IF THIS IS TUESDAY, IT MUST BE CHICKEN

IF THIS IS TUESDAY, IT MUST BE CHICKEN

OR
HOW TO ROTATE YOUR FOOD FOR BETTER HEALTH

by
NATALIE GOLOS
&
FRANCES GOLOS GOLBITZ
Foreword by Doris Rapp, M.D.

Keats Publishing, Inc. New Canaan, Connecticut

Grateful acknowledgment is made for permission to reprint the excerpts from *Coping With Your Allergies* by Natalie Golos and Frances Golos Golbitz with Frances Spatz Leighton. Copyright © 1979 by Frances Golos Golbitz. Reprinted by permission of Simon & Schuster, a division of Gulf and Western Company.

Library of Congress Cataloging in Publication Data

GOLOS, NATALIE
    If this is Tuesday, it must be chicken, or How to rotate your food for better health.

    Bibliography: p. 123.
    Includes index.
    1. Food allergy—Diet therapy.   2. Food allergy—
Diet therapy—Recipes.   I. Golbitz, Frances Golos.
II. Title.

RC596.G64   616.97′5   83-9439
                                 AACR2

ISBN 0-87983-339-4

Printed in the United States of America

Keats Publishing, Inc., 27 Pine Street
New Canaan, Connecticut 06840

CONTENTS

ACKNOWLEDGMENTS

I would like to thank the members of the Society for Clinical Ecology and also the Human Ecology Action League (HEAL) for their generous sharing of ideas.

Particular mention must be made for the help received from Jeannine Kantor and Vera Rea and especially from Jane Roller for her indispensable work on the food families.

A special note of thanks goes to my first three mentors: Drs. Eloise Kailin, Theron Randolph and Lawrence Dickey, and also to the four physicians who most recently have assisted and encouraged me: Drs. Doris Rapp, Phyllis Saifer, William Rea and Sidney Baker.

Natalie Golos

For my part, I would like to thank Glyn Nelson, Sally Pruit and Robert and Iris Ingram.

Joan Hixon Martin deserves special recognition for her assistance in proofreading.

My final thanks go to my husband, Herman, who continually makes a contribution to all our literary efforts, and to my young grandson, Ricky Golbitz, who designed the first cover of this book.

Frances Golos Golbitz

This book is dedicated to Dr. and Mrs. Theron Randolph whose concern for the patient resulted in their forming and nurturing the first ecologic support group.

FOREWORD

We are now on the brink of the realization that a growing number of people of every age, including infants, have a newly recognized 20th century illness called ecologic or environmental disease. Although many aspects of this illness were described in the 30s and 40s by Albert H. Rowe, M.D. and Theron Randolph, M.D., only recently have a growing number of physicians become aware of the major role foods and chemicals play in modern day medicine.

It is unfortunate that Natalie Golos developed totally incapacitating ecologic illness many years ago. However, because of her own tremendous personal struggle, and the insight and help given to her by Drs. Kailin and Randolph, she is able to share the pearls of her success with you in this book. Her previous book, *Coping With Your Allergies*, was written mainly to help those persons who had a complex ecologic illness, and it contains practical, sensible answers to the everyday food and chemical problems which face those who have severe ecologic health problems.

This new book is written primarily for those who are *not* incapacitated. It effectively explains exactly how a rotary diet is used to prevent food allergies in families prone to ecologic illness. It tells how to recognize offending foods and how to enjoy a varied diet so you can retain your good health or restore your previous feeling of well-being. This book anticipates the daily problems busy people face when attempting diets and realistically offers many choices and compromises, i.e., how to handle the desire to break or change a diet. The greatest asset of this book, however, is the simplicity and variety which it offers. Natalie Golos has used her imagination and wealth of knowledge to outline the essential recipes which will make the rotary diet workable and usable on a long term basis. Her suggestions make the diet not only tolerable but more pleasant.

In essence, this book simplifies and expands the rotary diet so that it is possible to enjoy a wide variety of foods. She will be revered by those who have found previous rotary diets a dreary, impossible challenge which robs them of the joy of eating. No longer can it be said that one does not know what to eat or that there is not enough to eat.

This book will also be helpful to many who may not associate their health problems with allergies. This includes the many people who are exhausted to the point of being unable to do their housework, nervous to the point of being unable to hold a job, irritable to the point of divorce, foggy-headed to the point of being unable to complete their education, and depressed to the point of suicide. Vast numbers of people are plagued with daily or intermittent unexplained muscle pain, joint aches, arthritis, abdominal pain, diarrhea, constipation, hypertension, heart disease, bizarre weakness, paralysis and seizures. Mothers feel inadequate and unworthy because no matter how hard they try, their children are always ill and no cause can be found. Amazing numbers of children are made to feel unloved, unwanted, bad and stupid at home and at school, because parents, teachers and physicians have failed to recognize the role foods and chemicals play in intolerable behavior, extreme fatigue, hyperactivity and inability to concentrate. Many children are embarrassed and punished daily because of passing gas, wetting the bed or soiling their underwear.

The manifestations of illness which I have just enumerated, of course, have multiple causes—but the one which is frequently overlooked is environmental illness. In some patients, the above medical problems stop when they find the role that unsuspected food or chemical offenders play in their illness.

This book has something to offer almost everyone. It will enable those with mild illness to stand alone. Those who have severely debilitating food and chemical illness do not just need this book. They *must have it*, as well as her other book. In addition, they need the personal care of an ecologically-oriented physician. Natalie Golos offers a way out when you are between a rock and a hard place. Once her method is mastered, you will have more time, more money and—most important—better health.

Natalie is a loving, caring and concerned person who graciously and altruistically is attempting to help others to cope better and more easily with their illness. Her book reflects her sympathetic and understanding nature. We are, indeed, fortunate to have a person with her expertise to help us. Bon appétit!

Doris J. Rapp, M.D., FAAA, FAAP
*Assistant Clinical Professor of Pediatrics
at the State University of New York
at Buffalo*

Author of *Allergies and the
Hyperactive Child* and *Allergies and
Your Family*

PREFACE

Perhaps you have been professionally diagnosed, by an allergist, as suffering from food allergies. Perhaps an internist has told you that the mysterious symptoms bothering you may be the result of allergies to food. Maybe you have merely read or heard something about the subject of food rotation and want more information about how to adjust your diet and eating practices.

Whatever the source and extent of your interest, the purpose of this book is to present a simplified approach to food rotation as a tool for prevention and management of food allergies.

For the convenience of the beginner, we have divided the approach to food allergies into five stages of procedure. These stages are meant to serve only as guidelines. You may find that you wish to practice some of the methods in Stages III and IV while you still consider yourself a candidate for Stage I.

Stage I is for those who are concerned about allergies but are reluctant to make extreme changes in eating habits.

Stage II is for those who have had good results from Stage I and are now more receptive to change.

Stage III is for those who know they have food allergies and have been advised to begin rotating their foods.

Stage IV is for the food-sensitive patients who do not have the additional problem of severe chemical sensitivity but have been advised to rotate all foods. It is also for chemically sensitive people who have stabilized their rotary diversified diet and are ready to begin rebuilding their adaptability (tolerance).

Stage V is the rotary-diversified diet as it is used for testing and treatment of severely allergic patients under the supervision of a physician.

THE FORMULA is the tool that makes rotation easier for everyone: for people in all five stages, for the professional who must plan individual diets for each patient, and for those who love to cook and bake and experiment with all kinds of recipes.

THE FORMULA helps you make frequent changes in the pattern of rotation without breaking your rotation.

Part I:
AN INTRODUCTION TO BETTER EATING HABITS

CHAPTER ONE

STAGE I: DIET MODIFICATION

Stage I is for those of you who are health oriented and wish to prevent allergies. It also addresses the vast majority of mildly allergic people who wish to prevent further trouble. Most important of all, it presents a beginning for those of you who know you or your children have food allergies but are reluctant to make extreme changes in your eating habits. Whatever the case may be, you can be as flexible as you choose. *DON'T TRY TO BE A ONE HUNDRED PERCENTER.* Don't drop the whole program because you can't do it all. Keep in mind that the smallest modification you make in your diet is a step in the right direction. As you go along you'll be surprised how a little knowledge can alter some of your eating habits without any effort. If you cook for a family, you can make major changes in your menu and no one will even notice the difference. Start by cutting down.

Cutting Down on Sugars

Any good nutrition program, especially in the case of an allergic person, strongly advises against sugar in any form (including raw turbinado, brown, beet, cane, maple, etc.). This applies especially to crystallized sugars. Your need decreases with your reduced intake. For snacks or desserts, adapt your taste to the natural sweetness of fresh fruit. When cooking, if the recipe calls for sugar, substitute maple syrup, honey, or a grain syrup such as malt, barley, corn, rice, sorghum or molasses and gradually cut down on these. The best substitutes are natural sweeteners like dates, figs, raisins, coconuts, etc.

Contrary to popular belief, raw turbinado sugar is not a substitute for white unrefined sugar; sugar is sugar regardless of its form (raw or refined). To compound the problem, there is an additional danger in the bacteria found in raw turbinado sugar.

3

Cutting Down on Prepackaged Foods

When you do buy them, read labels and select the product that states that it has *no* chemicals, additives or preservatives. However, please note that you cannot always trust the labels because, even when the food is pure, the packaging may not be. For example, the inside of cans is frequently treated with phenol, a preservative.

Cutting Down on Cooking

Unless your doctor has a reason for suggesting that you cook your foods, cut down on cooked vegetables and fruits. Gradually acquire a taste for raw vegetables such as broccoli, cauliflower, spinach. In the recipe sections you will find interesting combinations for salads. In Chapter 5, "Cooking Tips for the Allergic," you will find ideas for a wholesome approach to cooking methods.

Cutting Down on Junk Food

Substitute pure fruit juice for soft drinks and fruit drink mixes. Do not be fooled by advertising. When buying fruit drinks, avoid the products that are advertised as 10 percent fruit juice. It really means 90 percent is not. Consider what the remaining 90 percent does contain. Eat nuts, dried fruits, peanuts, roasted soy beans, sunflower seeds instead of candies. Make your own pop corn from pure popping corn (not one of the instant kinds). It is not only healthier, it's cheaper. Cut down on corn chips and potato chips but when you do buy them, buy the brand that uses pure safflower oil and has no preservatives or additives, and is packaged rather than canned.

Cutting Down on Refined Grains

The process of refining them removes most if not all of the nutrients. The manufactured nutrients they put back into the grain can be harmful to your health. Start using the whole grains, whole wheat, whole rice, etc.

Cutting Down on Salt

Even though salt is one ingredient that may be used every day, we earnestly recommend that you gradually reduce your intake until you have lost your dependence on it. Substitute herbs for seasoning.

CHAPTER TWO

STAGE II: THE COMMITMENT

This is essentially a "how to," not a "why" book. If, by now, the results from cutting down have not convinced you of the need to make a commitment, we suggest that you read Part I of *Coping with Your Allergies*,[1] and *An Alternative Approach to Allergies*.[2]

Elimination

In essence, part of Stage II is a continuation of Stage I, with greater concentration on omitting the worst offenders: refined sugars and grains, preservatives (especially BHT, BHA and nitrates), artificial colors and artificial flavors.

Flexibility

There are times when you are eating out that you are limited. Nevertheless, there is some choice. For example, you can order a baked potato instead of French fries which have probably been treated with preservatives to prevent discoloration. If you hunger for French fries, make them at home, using untreated oil and cutting down on or eliminating salt.

Seek Non-Professional Help

Now that you are really committed to improving your diet, seek the help of those who have experience with diets for the allergic. Join the HUMAN ECOLOGY ACTION LEAGUE (HEAL), an organization dedicated to education about clean food, clean water and clean air.[3] A local chapter will help you find local sources of good foods and can advise you about name brand availability in your area.

If there is no local chapter, your local health food store will know people with similar interests about food. Help organize these people and suggest that they ask the supermarket manager to

5

provide a special section that will have only those foods that are sugarless and free from perservatives and additives such as artificial colors and flavors. This will cut down on shopping time and simultaneously educate the local grocer who will help inform the food industry that there is a demand for more wholesome food.

Self-Education

Make a commitment to learn as much as you can about food allergies. In the beginning, we suggest you limit your reading to authors of books on clinical ecology, the field of medicine that studies man in relation to his environment (food, water and air).

Refer to Appendix D for a list of suggested readings. Most of these books should be available in your local library. If not, ask that they be ordered. Incidentally, this is another way of educating the public.

Having read the books, you will then be able to choose which ones to purchase for day-to-day reference.

Professional Help

If you are ill and the cause has not been found, do not despair. Despite what you may have been told, you probably do not have to learn to live with aches and pains. Many so-called hypochondriacs have found help by consulting a physician who understands "ecologic illness"—sensitivity to foods, drugs and chemicals. In the list of organizations (Appendix C), you will find the address of the Society for Clinical Ecology. They will help you locate such a doctor.

CHAPTER THREE

STAGE III: EASING INTO ROTATION

We are the last people to suggest that it is easy to change a lifelong pattern of eating. That is why it is easier to begin rotation at birth or at least in the very early years when habits and patterns are first being formed. Usually only the seriously ill are willing to make abrupt changes; in fact, they are willing to try anything.

Most others need to ease into rotation. You may be at this stage because your physician has told you that you have food allergies and you should begin rotating foods. You may be considering rotation because you accept the idea by deduction from your own experience or from reading about food allergies.

Some Reasons for Rotation

Many people have mild food allergies which are of clinical importance primarily because exposure to these foods never really stops; they are eaten so frequently that a cumulative effect results. A rotary diet gives you an opportunity to clear such foods from your system. This prevents those cumulative effects which cause varying degrees of illness.

Advantages of Rotation

Rotation preserves your tolerance for non-offending foods presently being eaten, tolerance being the ability to eat food without becoming ill. This technique of eating also serves to prevent the development of new allergies that often occur when you are over-exposed to any given food.

For an in-depth discussion of the value of rotating foods, read about the rotary diversified diet in *Coping With Your Allergies*[1] and *An Alternative Approach to Allergies*.[2]

7

Food Families

In Appendix A you will find charts of Food Families. It is important to be aware that foods come in families. If you are allergic to cucumber, you may also react to zucchini. Because they look alike, it is no surprise that they are both in the same family; however, it may not be so obvious that cantaloupe is also of that family and therefore a potential problem to those sensitive to cucumber or zucchini.

As you advance further in your education, you will learn much more about food families and rotation. However, this stage is designed only to ease into rotation. At the end of this chapter you will find a beginner's chart of foods divided into four days. Foods are then divided into categories: animal protein, vegetables and fruits. Here again, as you begin, it is worth repeating: *"DON'T TRY TO BE A 100 PERCENTER."* Don't disregard the entire idea of rotating if you don't want to do it completely. If you are not ready to be concerned with rotation of all foods, begin with your animal protein: meat, fish, fowl, etc.

From among the more familiar proteins listed in the chart, you could choose, for example, one or more of the following:

Day 1—Monday: Cheese, cod fish, haddock, milk or beef.
Day 2—Tuesday: Tuna fish, turkey or carp.
Day 3—Wednesday: Trout, perch, salmon, ham or pork (uncured).
Day 4—Thursday: Sole, flounder, halibut, eggs or chicken.

Rotating Vegetables and Fruits

When you are ready you can advance to rotating vegetables and fruits from the chart. You will find the variety pleasing to the palate. To make food preparation easier, Chapter 5, "Cooking Tips for the Allergic," will give you some short cuts for preparing these foods from scratch.

BEGINNER'S CHART

	Day 1, 5, 9, etc.	Day 2, 6, 10, etc.	Day 3, 7, 11, etc.	Day 4, 8, 12, etc.
ANIMAL PROTEIN	Crab, crayfish, lobster, prawn, shrimp. Cod, haddock. Ocean catfish. Herring, sardine. Catfish species. Beef (butter, cheese, kefir, milk, veal, yogurt) buffalo, goat, sheep (lamb, mutton).	Tuna, mackerel. White fish. Pike. Carp, chub. Frogs legs. Turtle. Dove, pigeon (squab). Turkey, turkey eggs.	Abalone, clam, cockle, mussel, oyster, scallop, snail, squid. All species of bass, all perch, all trout, croaker, grouper, salmon, sauger, walleye. Rabbit. Swine (bacon, ham, pork—uncured).	Swordfish. Flounder, halibut, sole, turbot. Duck, goose (eggs). Ruffed grouse (partridge). Chicken (eggs), pheasant, quail, guinea fowl. Squirrel.
VEGETABLES	Mushroom, truffle. Corn, bamboo shoots. Eggplant, sweet pepper, potato, tomato.	Malanga. Ñame, yam. Beet, chard, spinach. Yuca. Olive. Cucumber, pumpkin, squash, zucchini.	Chinese water chestnut. Carrot, celeriac (celery root), celery, parsley, parsnip. Sweet potato. Artichoke, dandelion, endive, Jerusalem artichoke, lettuce.	Asparagus, chives, garlic, leek, onion, shallot. Broccoli, brussels sprouts, cabbage, cauliflower, chinese cabbage, collards, kale, kohlrabi, mustard greens, radish, rutabaga, turnip, watercress. Alfalfa, all beans, all peas, peanut, soybean. Okra.
FRUIT	Avocado. Apple, crabapple, loquat, pear, quince. Acerola. Dried currant, grape, raisin. Pomegranate.	Banana, plantain. Custard apple, paw-paw. Apricot, cherry, peach, plum. Guava. Bearberry, blueberry, cranberry, huckleberry. Cantaloupe, melon, watermelon.	Date, coconut, Pineapple. Rhubarb. Currant, gooseberry. Blackberry, raspberry, strawberry. Litchi. Persimmon.	Fig. Grapefruit, kumquat, lemon, lime, muscat, orange, pummelo, tangelo, tangerine. Mango. Kiwi (Chinese gooseberry). Papaya.

CHAPTER FOUR

STAGE IV: FOOD ROTATION MADE EASY

When you are planning and cooking for the family, making rotation work for you can be a challenge. A child may "get a kick" out of a breakfast that consists of only nuts and fruit, but a lunch without bread may present problems. A teenager will welcome a snack of two big bowls of home-made popcorn but frown on giving up coke and chocolate bars. In our experience, the same holds true for adults.

We have two suggestions that have helped. First, include the entire family in the education. Have family reading sessions from our suggested reading list so that even the children can learn the why and how of prevention and good health as related to good eating habits.

The second suggestion is to have the entire family involved as a preventive procedure rather than singling out one member as the "sick" one. As the family improves their eating habits, you will soon notice the so-called "healthy" members remarking about their increased energy, their improved state of mind as well as the disappearance of minor, but not insignificant, irritation or discomfort.

A Word of Caution

We feel it important to remind you, at this point, that Stage IV is *not* for the patient with uncontrolled severe food and chemical sensitivities. Such patients must have Stage V guidance which is covered in depth in *Coping With Your Allergies*.[1]

The rotation plan that we are presenting in this book is to be used for prevention or for people with mild food sensitivities. It should be used by the severely allergic individual only after he has stabilized his diet or has his food allergies under control with the assistance of a doctor (using drops or injections).[2,4]

How to Use Stage IV

There are three ways to use Stage IV. The easiest way is to use the information exactly as it is provided in Chapters 7, 8, 9 and 10. Chapter 7 presents the Table of Contents, the food chart, the menus, and recipes for days 1, 5 and 9 of three four-day cycles. The next three chapters follow the same pattern for the other rotating days. To see the total picture, refer to the four pages of Appendix B.

The other two ways to use Stage IV are procedures following a formula that teaches you how to make changes in your rotation pattern. *DO NOT CHANGE ANY FOOD FROM ONE DAY TO ANOTHER UNTIL YOU HAVE READ THE FORMULA AT THE END OF THIS CHAPTER.* At that point you will find an explanation of the number system that simplifies making changes. Until then, ignore the numbers. By following the four chapters, you will be sure that you are following a four-day rotation.

Varying Degrees of Rotation

Some clinical ecologists teach that you can eat any food (or member of that food family) all day long provided none of them is repeated again during that four-day cycle: cherries, almonds and peaches all day long. A second approach restricts the intake of any food to one meal in the four-day cycle, but permits eating any related foods (members of the same family) during that same day: almonds with breakfast, cherries with lunch, peaches with dinner. A stricter approach limits an entire food family to one meal during the whole four-day cycle: almonds, cherries and peaches all at one meal and not repeated for the rest of the four-day cycle.

With any of the above procedures you can use our recipes and food charts. You may wish to modify some of the menus for the more restrictive measures. If your doctor uses some other procedure, he or she can easily show you how to use our charts to conform with his/her method.

Nutritional Requirements

Once you and your family have adjusted to the idea of rotation you may wish to change the order of your rotation. Before you do, you should know the facts we considered as we prepared our rotation. Our first objective in dividing foods over a period of four days was good nutrition. If you eat whole unprocessed foods as

11

recommended in Part I you will obtain a proper intake of minerals, vitamins, amino acids and essential fatty acids. You do not need to be concerned about a balanced diet of individual days, so long as food consumed over the four-day period meets the nutritional requirements.

However, as much as possible, daily nutrition was a very important consideration. Each day includes protein, fruit, a green leafy vegetable and a yellow vegetable. Oranges and other citrus fruits are on a different day from tomato (the Potato Family) because these are the two families highest in vitamin C. Similarly we separated carrots and apricots, two foods highest in vitamin A.

The basic plan ensures that each day includes some type of seeds and nuts, oils and fats, herbs and spices, beverages and a starch for sauces and puddings. Although we firmly believe that you can learn to like foods without sweeteners, we have included one for each day, with the recommendation that you reduce the amount each time until you have lost your dependence on sweets.

Rotating Animal Food Families

In order to make your own changes there is something you must understand about the structure of Animal Food Families. They are first divided into categories: mollusks, crustaceans, fish, birds and mammals. These categories are then subdivided into families. Refer to Appendix B. Notice that you have a choice of fish for every single day. This can be done because fish are divided into many different families. The same holds true for fowl and red meats. If you are planning for meat two days within the four-day cycle it is advisable to have a day between them. Notice that you can have beef on Day 1 and pork on Day 3 because they are different families. However, you could not have beef on Day 1 and lamb on Day 3 because they are the same family. Of course the best possible plan is to have a red meat on one day, a fowl on another, a fish on another and a crustacean on another. All of these contingencies are incorporated into our plan. That is why, to make it even easier for you to follow this rotation, we have recipes and suggested menus that correspond to each day's rotation.

Confusion in Names

In the fish family, names can cause confusion. Perch is an example of this: silver perch belongs to the Croaker Family; white perch, to the Bass Family. Because they are easily confused even by fish market people and a wrong choice could upset your rotation we are treating them as one family and putting them all on one day.

This same problem exists within the plant food families. Arrowroot may come from the Arrowroot Family, the Banana Family, or one of six other sources. Because health food store personnel usually don't know the source, we treat all types of arrowroot almost as one family, putting them all on one day.

Taste Appeal

For taste appeal, whenever possible we tried to retain customary combinations like cranberries and turkey on the same day. On another day we have mustard, eggs and lemons, the ingredients for mayonnaise. On Day 1 both yeast and grains are included so that bread can be made.

Incidentally, yeast and cheese, a mold product, belong to the same family, so cheese also appears on Day 1. Because cheese is also a milk product, it must be on the same day as beef and goat (of the same family). This will give you an idea of the many factors we took into consideration.

THE FORMULA

There are so many variables in planning a rotary diversified diet, that it is virtually impossible for any book, including our former three books, to present one plan that can be universally used. That is why it was necessary to devise a system that could be so flexible that it could meet anyone's needs. It may help you to understand the scope and versatility of the rotary diet if you know the complications involved in developing our formula.

A formula must consider the state of health of the individual: a healthy member of a family prone to allergies; the mildly sensitive individual; the patient with food allergies; the patient with multiple sensitivities . . . food, inhalants, chemicals, etc.; or, finally, the patient in varying degrees of recovery.

A formula must take into account the purpose of the diet: prevention of allergies, diagnosis (testing for allergies), treatment or maintenance. A formula must accommodate the individual's food allergy enabling him/her to use it with ease as dietary needs change.

A formula must accommodate the different approaches of doctors so their medical assistants will find it easier to plan all the individual diets of their patients and to teach patients to make necessary changes.

Reason for Changes

There could be circumstances under which you would want to make permanent changes. You would do so if you were allergic to one or more foods of every vegetable family listed for a particular day. As an example, say that you were so allergic to mushrooms, corn and potatoes that you would want to avoid every food in their families. That would leave you without a vegetable for that day unless you made a permanent change.

Another reason for a permanent change would be a situation where you had all of the vegetables you prefer on one day and all those you dislike on another day. You would want to make certain changes to avoid that.

The most important and exciting change, however, is the temporary one that gives you such a variety that without breaking your rotation you can use any recipe that can be cooked "from scratch."

How to Change

To make any change easily all you need is an explanation of the numbers we have given to all of the food families and the ways that we are using them.

Turn to Appendix A to find these numbers as they relate to the food families. There is no botanical reason for the numbers, and you will not find them in any book on botany. They are listed as a convenience to the reader to make it easier to plan your rotation. Each food is listed in two ways, alphabetically with its corresponding food family number, and numerically with all of the foods in one family listed together. The first entry under C of the alphabetical list is the word "cabbage" preceded by the number "36." When you turn to List #2, the numerical list of food families, you find that "36" is the Mustard Family and so you discover all the foods that belong to the same family that cabbage does.

These numbers are repeated any time a member of the family appears on a list. This simplifies changing any food from one day to another.

Now turn to Appendix B. At the top of each day's chart you will find a list of the numbers of every food family included for that day. You will also find the corresponding number before each family.

Suppose you want to change corn from Day 1 to another day. Check the chart to find the number for corn. It happens to be six. Everything identified as Number Six has to be moved with the corn. You would have to transfer the following:

From Vegetables: 6-Corn, bamboo shoots.
From Fats and Oils: 6-Corn oil, rice oil.
From Miscellaneous: 6-Barley, millet, oat, rice, rye.
From Sweeteners: 6-Grain syrups: barley, corn, malt, molasses and sorghum.
From Herbs and Spices: 6-Lemongrass.

As you change your charts, do not forget to remove the number 6 from the top of the page where you find the numbers of all the foods used on Day 1. Then add 6 to the list of numbers for the new day. This will keep your own charts up to date.

Bear in mind that the recipes apply to the numbering as we presented it. You will find the same number system throughout the book.

Easy Temporary Changes

As you read about and begin to make temporary changes, it may seem very involved. After a few times it will become second nature and as easy to do as any meal you ever planned.

It is easier to make temporary changes of foods when they are on days adjacent to each other—days 1 and 2, 2 and 3, 3 and 4 or 4 and 5, Day 5 being a repetition of Day 1. Whenever you wish to make temporary changes it is wise to plan ahead, checking your charts on the first day of any rotation cycle.

Suppose you decide to serve maple syrup with your buckwheat pancakes on Day 3. In checking your charts, you will find maple syrup must be moved from Day 2 to Day 3. Follow your rotation as usual only omitting the Maple family (50) from Day 2. On the next cycle return to the original rotation, eating the syrup on Day 2.

If you want to add onions to the Day 1 spaghetti sauce recipe (Chapter 7), check your chart and you will find that onions of the

Lily family (11) are included on Day 4. Follow your rotation as indicated on Day 1, 2 and 3 but then, on Day 4, omit the Lily family because you are switching onions from Day 4 to Day 1 of the next cycle.

CAUTION: *If you are highly susceptible to certain foods or if foods are being moved more than one day, it would be wise to omit the switched food family for two full cycles, once before and once after they are switched.*

Changes: Permanent or Temporary?

There may be times that you need to choose between a permanent change and a temporary change. This can best be illustrated with a peanut bread recipe taken from *Coping With Your Allergies*.[1] We did not include the recipe in Chapter 10 (Day 4), because the cream of tartar in the baking powder upsets the rotation. Cream of tartar belongs to the Grape Family (52) which is included on Day 1 (See Appendix B).

PEANUT BREAD

1 cup peanut flour	1 egg
½ teaspoon salt	¾ cup water
3 teaspoons baking powder	2 tablespoons honey
2 teaspoons peanut oil	

Preheat oven to 350°F. Sift flour before measuring. Mix dry ingredients. Combine honey, oil and water and then add beaten egg. Blend with dry ingredients. Bake in 4″ × 7″ × 2″ pan for 40 minutes.

To be sure your baking powder is pure, make your own. For instructions see Chapter 5, "Cooking Hints for the Allergic." Caution: *Recipes seldom mention that cream of tartar is one ingredient in baking powder.*

Any time you want to serve this peanut bread on Day 4, be sure to omit the Grape Family from Day 1 of your next rotation. In fact you may want to change the Grape Family permanently to Day 4. Before you do, consider all the reasons for and against.

First check Chapter 7 to see why we placed the Grape Family on Day 1 instead of Day 4. See how many recipes require the combinations of grains and baking powder: biscuits, crackers, muffins,

16

breads, cookies, etc. If you were to make a permanent change to Day 4, you would be eliminating all of those recipes from Day 1.

You might consider a permanent change if you were allergic to all grains and were avoiding them anyhow. Also, it is tempting to make a permanent change because Day 4 has so many combinations that make good sandwiches: chicken salad, tofu with alfalfa and chives, egg salad, and then, there are always peanut butter sandwiches.

As a good compromise, you could leave the plan as it is, making the temporary change to Day 4 as often as you wish to make bread. When you do, if you wish to have bread on Day 1 of that rotation, be sure that you use a recipe that calls for yeast and not baking powder. Also, remember to avoid other members of the Grape Family, i.e., grapes, raisins, etc., on Day 1 of that cycle.

CHAPTER FIVE

COOKING HINTS FOR THE ALLERGIC

The reason prepackaged foods are so popular is, of course, that they save time. It is possible to reduce the time it takes to prepare food from scratch through short-cuts that we would like to share with you. As you get more involved with it, you will soon learn how to devise your own time-saving procedures. In addition, it will benefit you to learn the cooking methods that minimize the loss of nutrients and some of the substitutions used by people with food allergies.

Baking Powder: Since it is difficult to know what ingredients are added to commercial baking powder, it is wise to prepare your own using cream of tartar (of the Grape Family, 52) and baking soda. When you are making your own, notice that it takes one teaspoon cream of tartar added to ½ teaspoon baking soda to equal only 1 teaspoon baking powder.

Cereal is much tastier if soaked overnight and cooked in a double boiler. The same is true of rice and dried beans and peas.

Cured and Smoked Foods: Avoid meat or fish that are cured, smoked or treated in a similar way.

Grain Syrup comes in different forms: barley syrup, corn syrup, malt syrup, molasses, sorghum grain syrup and a combination of two or three. In most cases, the texture is so thick, you have to thin the syrup before you can add it to a recipe. To do this combine the syrup with heated liquid (whatever liquid the recipe calls for).

If the recipe does not call for liquid, boil 2 tablespoons of water in a saucepan; gradually add syrup and more water until the syrup has reached the consistency of honey. You must use it immediately or the syrup will begin to solidify again.

Legumes (beans, peas, etc.) should always be cooked or sprouted. We have learned this from Dr. Alsoph Corwin, Chemistry Profes-

18

sor Emeritus from Johns Hopkins University. According to Dr. Corwin, legumes contain a group of mildly toxic substances called lectins, which can present a danger if taken over a long period of time. However, their toxicity is destroyed by cooking or sprouting.

Peanut Butter: When you buy peanut butter, be sure that it is pure—no additives, no preservatives, no sugar, no salt. If it does contain vegetable oil, be sure that it is pure peanut oil.

Nothing equals making your own. It is usually cheaper and always safer. See Chapter 6 for recipe for nut butter.

Raw Fruits and Vegetables: Cooking, especially with high heat, destroys many nutrients. Therefore, as previously mentioned, unless your doctor has recommended otherwise, eat your foods raw whenever possible. Our recipes for cooked foods such as the baked apples are suggested for occasional use. Raw fruit is more nutritious.

Gradually develop a taste for raw vegetables, too. Begin by introducing into your salads vegetables that your family has always eaten cooked, such as zucchini, asparagus, broccoli and cauliflower. Don't be afraid to try new approaches. Many vegetables that have always been eaten cooked actually taste better raw particularly when added to a salad.

For example, on Day 4 add raw cauliflower to your cabbage salad with mayonnaise or sesame cream or some other salad dressing. Later you may want to try cauliflower as an appetizer with a dip of tahini (sesame seed butter), fig nut salad dressing or sesame cream. The recipes are found in Chapter 10. In time, you will enjoy eating it plain as you would an apple or orange.

In a similar way, you can acquire a taste for almost any raw vegetable, or for sprouts which have exceptional food value.

SPROUTS

Seeds That May Be Sprouted: Alfalfa, beans, cereal grain, red clover, cress, fenugreek, lentils, mung beans, oats, parsley, dried peas, radish, rye and almost any other seed that will grow.

Why Sprout Seeds? Seeds when sprouted are more easily digested. Patients allergic to some seeds can sometimes tolerate them when sprouted. The nutrient value increases with sprouting.

Methods for Growing Sprouts: 1) Select good quality seeds—those not sprayed or treated with chemicals or preservatives. 2) A one or two quart wide-mouthed jar is simplest and most inexpensive to use. A piece of cotton gauze or a fine stainless steel screen should be held in place over the mouth of the jar by a rubber band or a canning ring. For a one-quart jar: use one level tablespoon of alfalfa seeds or 2 level tablespoons of mung beans (or other large seeds). Be sure to remove all broken or cracked seeds or they will rot and spoil sprouts.

Put in jar and cover with several inches of lukewarm water. Place net or cheesecloth over jar and secure with rubber band. Soak seeds overnight in a dark cupboard for about five hours. Drain and rinse well. Lay jar on its side in a fairly dark place for the first couple of days. However, be sure to rinse with lukewarm water 2–3 times daily. Flood jar and drain well each time. *Rinsing is the key to good sprouts.* As the seeds germinate they produce heat and waste. Thus, they must be faithfully cooled and washed at least mornings and evenings to produce a tasty crop.

Rule: Keep them warm and moist all the time, but not wet. Cold delays growth. Too much heat encourages molding. When leaves begin to show (about the 4th day), allow light on jar. Place near window for more vitamin A and chlorophyll. When two green leaves have opened out fully, sprouts are at the height of their value and ready to use.

One-fourth cup mung beans will give you about two cups of bean sprouts.

When To Eat Sprouts: Alfalfa sprouts taste best when 1 to 2 inches long. Mung beans are best when 1½ to 3 inches long. Wheat sprouts are most delicious when the sprout is the length of the seeds. Lentil sprouts are edible within 36 hours and should be used when about 1 inch long. Sunflower seed sprouts are best when no longer than the seed. Pea and soybean sprouts are good short or long. When sprouts have developed to the desired stage, put into a glass jar in the refrigerator. They will keep for several days if properly covered, but never keep them longer than one week. Alfalfa sprouts take about five days or so to develop; mung beans, about 4 or 5 days. Wheat and lentil sprouts are ready in about 2 days.

Alfalfa Sprouts: These should never be cooked. Snack on them raw. Mix a handful with a favorite spread, tahini (sesame butter), mayonnaise or tofu. Add to salads, soup or stew just before serving. Excellent for sandwiches—in place of lettuce and a lot cheaper.

Lentil Sprouts: Lentil sprouts are good when added to soups just before serving. They may be prepared plain, with herbs, diced onions or any seasoning of the day.

Mung Bean Sprouts, one of the highest vegetable protein foods, taste like fresh pod peas when eaten raw. Add to omelets or soups of the day.

STEAMING FISH AND SEAFOOD

Frying and broiling should be avoided as much as possible—they are not healthy cooking methods. Steaming is preferred. It can be done easily in the oven by placing a stainless steel baking rack in a covered roasting pan with water covering the bottom of the pan up to but not touching the fish. Do not overcook your fish. Test it within 5 to 8 minutes, depending on the thickness of the fish. When you can flake it off with a slight pierce of the fork, the fish is ready to eat.

Use the water left over at the bottom of the pan to make a sauce using a little oil and some of the herbs in your rotation plan for that day.

To save time and to decrease the time that the fish is exposed to heat, use boiling water to cover the bottom of the pan and place in a preheated oven.

STEAMING MEAT OR FOWL

Use the same process you use for steaming fish. For large roasts and fowl we have found that they can bake in the oven at 250°F. overnight and be ready for breakfast. See introduction to Part II for a discussion of unconventional menus.

STEAMING VEGETABLES

When you do cook vegetables, the healthiest and easiest way is to prepare them in a stainless steel steamer basket. Nutrients and the flavor remain in the food instead of ending up in the water. Steam only until just barely fork tender.

Vegetable peeling has great value. If, however, you don't like the peel (or skin), it can be removed more easily after steaming and with less waste of the vegetables and of the nutrition. A potato examined under a microscope reveals that the cells closest to the peel have the greatest concentration of protein.

With raw vegetables, like cucumbers, begin by leaving some of the skin on and gradually increase the amount until you have educated your taste buds to enjoy the skin, the most wholesome part.

WARNING: MOLD ALLERGY

Mold on food skins can cloud the picture of food allergies. You may test negative to provocative testing[4] by your doctor but react to the food when you eat it at home. This means that you could be reacting not to the food but to the mold on the food. For an explanation of provocative testing, see *Allergies and the Hyperactive Child*[4] and *Allergies and Your Family*[6] by Doris Rapp, M.D. She discusses in depth the different types of food tests.

It is necessary to deal with mold on food according to the degree of sensitivity. Some patients can manage by wearing a mask and washing the vegetables thoroughly. Others need to have someone else do the vegetable washing for them. More severely sensitive persons need to have someone wash, peel and discard the peel from these mold-type vegetables. This applies especially to root vegetables, those that mature underground, such as yams, carrots, potatoes, etc.

If you are sensitive to molds avoid using dried foods such as dried fruits, dried herbs, etc. Use only fresh or frozen.

It is very easy to grow your own herbs. However, if you prefer to buy them, buy in large quantities at the height of the season. Wash them and place them on a cotton or linen towel. Pat them dry. Cut them into ½" snippings, using the leaves and the finer stems. Place on a cookie sheet and freeze. After several hours, remove from the cookie sheet, place in a glass jar or cellophane bag and return to the freezer for storage. This makes it possible to use in as small a quantity as needed.

Three herbs that work well with the above procedure are dill, tarragon and mint. This should work as well with chives.

Chemical Sensitivity: Even though you are not allergic to it, there is another reason that you could be reacting to a specific food. The cause could be the chemicals in the foods or the chemicals that were used to grow the foods. For a comprehensive discussion, refer to *Coping With Your Allergies*.[1] The index will direct you to sections covering "Food Sensitivities" and "Organic Foods."

Time and Money Savers

Fast Food: Cooking with a crock pot is a great time saver. The night before, wash and season your meat. When you awaken, put it into your crock pot on high for up to an hour. Before you leave the house be sure to turn it back to low.

When you get home, it is ready to eat. If you wish, you can even put the vegetables into the crock pot with your meat. The slow cook method is not only a convenience; it is said to be healthier.

As you progress with the program you will find many other ways to save time as well as money. One way is to buy when prices are low. Buy, cook and freeze in large quantities. For an in-depth discussion of these procedures for the allergic, and for other ideas, refer to *Coping With Your Allergies*,[1] especially the chapters "Cooking Hints," "Cooking in Quantity" and "Substitutions."

CHAPTER SIX

MAKING ROTATION WORK

For rotation of multiple food meals there are two simple approaches to use: fit the recipe to the foods, or fit the foods to the recipe.

The following example (#1) illustrates the first approach: building a recipe around the foods allowed on a particular day. For this example, we chose vegetable salads because they lend themselves to the widest range of choice and personal taste.

Examples #2 through #14 illustrate the second principle, selecting the foods according to the recipe. These are basic recipes which you can alter to fit almost any day.

Example #1: VEGETABLE SALADS

Make them as simple or as varied as you wish. However, always try to include a leafy green vegetable and/or sprouts.

If you are trying to ease the family into more simple fare limiting the number of food families per meal, use vegetables from the same family.

One-Food Family: Day 3, you can use lettuce, Jerusalem artichoke, endive and sunflower seeds. You can even use an oil from this same family (sunflower or safflower), and an herb such as tarragon.

Two-Food Families: From Day 4, cabbage, cauliflower and radishes make a delicious combination. Add sesame seeds and oil, and you have only two families.

Four-Food Families: If you wish to make it more elaborate but still limit families, you could make mayonnaise with sesame seed oil, mustard (same family as cabbage) and introduce only two new families (lemon and egg). Without increasing the number of families, you could then add chopped egg and diced cold leftover chicken. The salad could serve as a very filling and satisfying main course. Without increasing the number of food families, you could adhere

24

to the conventional pattern of eating by serving grapefruit as your appetizer and oranges as your dessert still using only four families.

Changing Pattern: By adding one more family, the Lily Family (11), you could serve asparagus as your vegetable, a side dish portion of the salad, and baked chicken and chicken soup flavored with garlic or onion.

Substitution: One more idea illustrates how you can play around with food families all on the same day, still working within your rotation. For the above salad omit the sesame seeds. Substitute peanut oil for the sesame seed oil to make your mayonnaise. Now you can really prepare a banquet. Because you are now using the legume family (peanuts), you could add alfalfa sprouts and/or cold cooked beans to your salad. With your chicken soup, you could serve noodles made with peanut starch. For dessert you could serve carob cookies with your oranges. (See Recipes Day 4— Chapter 10.)

You can follow this pattern any day of the cycle using the foods of that day.

Example #2: DRIED FRUITS OF THE DAY

One way of using dried fruit is to steam it. Add enough water (spring or distilled) so that the pot will not boil dry in 10 to 15 minutes. Cover tightly and steam 10–15 minutes or more if not yet tender. They can be eaten as is or stuffed with other fruit or nuts of the day.

Example #3: FISH OF THE DAY

Although there are specific recipes for certain days, fish can be served any day of the rotation using the ingredients of the day.

BAKED FISH

3 lbs. of fillet of fish of the day
4–6 cups mixed vegetables of the day

1 cup water
2 tablespoons herb of the day
salt to taste

Preheat oven to 350°F. Pour one cup of boiling water into baking dish. Add vegetables. Place fish on top of vegetables. Sprinkle fish with salt and herbs. Bake until fish flakes easily with a fork. If water needs to be added before fish is done, be sure it is boiling water.

Steamed Fish or Seafood: See Chapter 5, "Cooking Hints for Steaming Fish." Serve the fish plain or with an oil/herb dressing or a garnish or dressing found in recipes of the day.

GOOD COMBINATIONS:

Day 1: Cod, haddock, shrimp or lobster with avocado dressing or rice oil or corn oil seasoned with bay leaf, basil, sage, savory or a combination of these.

Day 2: Carp, chub, whitefish or pike with almond oil, apricot oil or olive oil seasoned with allspice or with olive oil dressing.

Day 3: Bass, perch, trout, croaker or walleye with safflower oil seasoned with kelp, dill or tarragon.

Day 4: Flounder, halibut, sole or turbot with peanut oil or sesame oil seasoned with chives.

Example #4: FRUIT BUTTER

Remove seeds and peeling from any fruit of the day and cut into quarters. Small fruit such as berries can be used whole. Lightly grease your crock pot with oil of the same family as the fruit used, or any other oil of the day. Do not fill the crock pot more than one inch from the top.

If desired you may add an herb of the day (about 1 teaspoon depending on taste). Allow to simmer on low, 24 hours or longer, until thickened to the consistency of apple butter.

Optional: Sweeten to taste just before using, with sweetener of the day. Some tasty combinations are:

Day 1: Apple or pear with cinnamon.

Day 2: Blueberry with maple syrup or ginger, cherry with banana and/or ginger, peach with banana.

Day 3: Blackberry, raspberry or strawberry with nutmeg, coconut and/or date sugar.

To can fruit butter, fill ½ pint or pint-sized sterilized Mason jars. Place on rack in pan of boiling water. Be sure that water is about 1 inch above the jars. Cover pan and boil for 10 minutes. Butter thickens as it stands.

Example #5: NUTS OF THE DAY

One pound in the shell yields about ½ pound of nut meats. To shell hardshell nuts more easily (butternuts, Brazil nuts, filberts, walnuts, pecans): pour boiling water over nuts and let stand 15 minutes. Drain and shell.

Example #6: NUT OR SEED BUTTER

*1 cup nuts or seeds of the
 day*

*1 tablespoon oil of the day
herb of the day* (optional)

Grind or blend repeatedly until fine and smooth. Store in the refrigerator.

This is a recipe that can be used any day of the rotation as long as you use the food listed for that day. Obviously you should use almond oil with almonds, sunflower oil with sunflower seeds, sesame oil with sesame seeds. In other cases, select the mildest oil to add to your seeds or nuts. For example, on Day 2, when you are using pumpkin seeds, you have a choice of apricot, almond or olive oil. Since olive oil has such a strong, distinctive taste and odor, you would be wise to select the less obtrusive apricot or almond oil.

Example #7: NUT OR SEED FRUIT CHEESE

*1 pound dried, seeded fruit
of the day*

*½ pound nuts or seeds of the
day*

Grind dried fruit and nuts (or seeds) very fine. Mix well. Pack firmly in glass baking dish so that mixture is ¼ to 1 inch thick.

Cover and let stand 2 or 3 days to dry. Cut with sharp knife into little strips. Roll in additional ground nuts or seeds. (You may want to combine several fruits and nuts of the day using the same proportion for each, by weight.)

Example #8: NUT OR SEED FRUIT PIE

For the Crust: Use any nut or seed of the day. Meal can be made by placing nuts or seeds ½ cup at a time into a blender. For soft nuts (like cashews) use chop speed; for hard nuts, grind speed. (For ease of use, if you have an Osterizer, use an Oster jar. If the Ball brand of Mason jar with narrow mouth fits tightly on the blade, it can be substituted.) A food processor, when available, is the fastest method.

The oil of the nuts causes the nuts nearest the blade to lump together; separate these from the dry nuts in the center, using them for the bottom crust and saving the drier nuts for the top crust. The oily nuts may need an additional teaspoon or two of oil for the crust. (This depends on how oily the nut used is and how long you kept it in the blender.)

Grease pie plate lightly with oil and press oily nuts or seeds into plate covering bottom and sides to ¼ of an inch thickness. (Eight heaping teaspoons provide a generous crust for a small deep dish pie; about 2 cups are needed for a nine inch pie.) Some people prefer a thinner crust. Add oil to part of the nutmeal and then press oily nuts first with spoon and then firmly with thumbs. You must judge amount of oil that will be needed and if too much oil was used, add more nutmeal. If you like it thicker, you can always add more nuts or seeds later.

For the Filling:

2 *cups liquid of the day*
2 *tablespoons starch of the day*
  optional: *fresh or frozen fruit of the day*
  optional: *1 tablespoon sweetener of the day*

The liquid can be any juice of the day (except citrus for which you need a different recipe), any stewed fruit and/or frozen fruit which has been allowed to defrost and soak in its own juice. The starch can be any starch of the day: arrowroot, tapioca, cornstarch, potato starch, rice flour, rye flour, artichoke flour, etc. The first four are the best thickeners for fillings.

Pour liquid over starch, mixing thoroughly. Heat at medium temperature, stirring constantly, being very careful not to burn. As soon as it thickens, remove from heat. (A double boiler is the best way to heat filling.) Tapioca is one starch that thickens after it is removed from the heat.

After filling has cooled, spoon it over bottom crust leaving room for fruit if you are using any. Cover filling with crushed dry nuts, seeds and coconut or meringue. Place cover over pie plate to keep dry nuts from browning before bottom crust.

Place in oven preheated to 400°F. for 20–40 minutes (or until bottom crust is lightly browned).

The following are tasty combinations:

	DAY 1	DAY 2	DAY 3
Crust:	Pecans	Almonds	Filberts
Liquid:	Apple juice	Cherry, apricot or peach juice	Strawberry juice
Oil:	Walnut, rice or corn oil	Almond oil	Safflower oil
Starch:	Potato starch or corn starch	Arrowroot starch	Agar-Agar
Sweetener:	Partially cooked sweet apples or grain syrup (cinnamon optional)	Cherries or peaches, maple syrup	Strawberries, date sugar or coconut

On Day 3, follow directions on package for agar-agar (sometimes called agar).

Example #9: NUT OR SEED FRUIT PUDDING

For a simple variation of the pie of Example #8, use the pie filling recipe of the day. After the filling cools and just before serving, add chopped nuts of the day or fruit of the day.

Example #10: NUT OR SEED MILK

1 part nuts of the day   *1 part water or juice of the day*

Combine and soak 24 to 48 hours. Drain liquid (saving it). Blend nuts on low speed until smooth as you would nut or seed butter, using liquid of soaked nuts instead of oil. When smooth, gradually add rest of liquid. If it is still too thick you can add more liquid.

Optional: Flavor with an herb of the day.
Optional: Sweeten to taste.

NOTE: Some people prefer to strain the milk and use the leftovers on recipes calling for nuts or seeds.

Example #11: NUT OR SEED/STARCH PANCAKE (Blender)

> 1 cup starch of the day
> 1 cup seeds or nuts of the day
> Liquid as needed (water or nut milk of the day)

Blend dry mixture at low speed adding liquid, gradually increasing the speed.

Note: Because there is no leavening, the pancake will be flatter than usual. Therefore, the batter should be thicker than usual. As you experiment for the right consistency, remember that it is easier to add liquid than dry mixture. To grease the griddle, when possible, use the oil made from the seed or nut used. Example: sunflower oil with sunflower seeds, almond oil with almonds. Otherwise use any oil of the day.

Example #12: POPSICLE OF THE DAY

> 1 pint of any juice or combination of juice of the day

Fill an ice cube tray with juice and place in freezer. Wait until juice begins to solidify (time depends on the type of juice). Put wooden uncolored, unflavored toothpick into each cube of juice.

Wait about 24 hours until they are thoroughly solid. Remove from tray, place in glass jar. Children, and adults, can enjoy unlimited popsicles in a very wholesome way.

Example #13: SOUP OF THE DAY

A little imagination, a little meat and bones of a mammal or fowl of the day, a few teaspoons of some herbs of the day will give you a hot soup for any cold day.

Variations: Add two or three vegetables of the day for a very filling soup that can be a meal in itself.

Example #14: SUBSTITUTE SLUSHIES AND SLURPIES

These two are commercial drinks popular among teenagers. Depending on the locality and store, they usually consist of flavored, colored and sugared drinks that have been partially frozen so they are like crushed ice.

To make a healthful substitute for slushies, fill an ice cube tray with any fruit juice of the day. Partially freeze. Remove the dividers and stir frequently. Serve when it reaches the consistency of crushed ice.

Variation: Add Perrier water (to give it the carbonated effect), and an herb and/or sweetener of the day, and you will have a wholesome substitute for slurpies.

Part II:
ROTATION: A TASTY
AND NUTRITIOUS APPROACH

By now it must be obvious that this approach to recipes and menus is very different from your usual cookbook. Because foods cannot be repeated daily, conventional recipes will not always be available every day of a basic plan. Therefore, this part is divided into four chapters, each chapter devoted to one day of the four-day rotation cycle.

As if they were four different cookbooks, each chapter contains its own table of contents which guides you to the list of foods for that day and suggested menus and recipes that follow that food list. Each table of contents must be different because some days have no breads; some, no dairy products; others, no cakes or biscuits. To reduce the margin for error, each chapter shows the numbers of the days on which it is to be followed.

Because our menus have been prepared to help you in the transition period, we have listed suggestions which more closely conform to conventional meals. Gradually you may become accustomed to meals that consist of only one course of substantial quantity. Thus you might eat one-half pound of fish for breakfast, three papayas for lunch or one pound of broccoli for dinner.

As you check the menus, remember that you can mix or match them, omitting meals that take too much time, repeating the favorite ones or those which are easiest and least expensive. These are merely suggestions to get you started. You may wish to eat breakfast from one menu and lunch from another . . . as long as you stick to the suggestions in the same chapter for any one day of the rotation.

Careful observation will show you that only the first suggested menu of each day represents the restricted approach for those people who do not wish to repeat any food family for more than one meal in any given cycle. For everything suggested in the menus, you will find a recipe either in the recipe section for that day or in Chapter 6. Also, in these two places you will find ideas for recipes not included in the suggested menus.

Salt and Sweeteners: Manufactured foods are so saturated with salt and sweeteners that the average consumer finds it difficult to do without them. Therefore with great reluctance we have included these unwholesome ingredients in our recipes with the suggestion that you gradually decrease the amount you use. In time you will decrease your dependence on them and develop an appreciation for nature's flavors.

35

Unused Food Families: Appendix A lists 137 families. If you carefully check the numbers used in the food charts of Appendix B, you discover there are many families that were not used. These foods fall in different classes:

a) Plants that are not edible: 15-orris, 38-yellow dye, 67-chicle.
b) Food and food factions that are not recommended: 5-gin, 12-tequila, 21-black and white pepper, 57-tea, 76-coffee, etc. If you do use them occasionally, make sure that it is on a rotation basis.
c) Another class of foods consists of vegetables, mostly leafy green vegetables that add to a salad. Some of them grow wild; others are available only in certain parts of the country. Check into them and fit them into your charts on a day you can use an extra vegetable: 29-New Zealand spinach, 30-pigweed, 37-caper, 42-oxalis, 43-nasturtium, 78-fetticus, commonly known as corn salad.
d) The fourth class not in the charts consists of animal protein, not available in many places. Check Appendix A if you wish to add any of the following to your charts: *84, 85, 86, 89, 90, 92, 93, 94, 95, 97, 99, 101, 104, 105, 108, 110, 116, 118, 119* and *128*.

CHAPTER SEVEN

MENUS AND RECIPES FOR DAYS

1,

TABLE OF CONTENTS

5,

9,

ETC.

FOOD CHART FOR DAYS 1, 5, 9, ETC.

Food Families Used:	2, 6, 22, 34, 35, 40a, 42, 46, 52, 61, 62, 73, 74, 82, 87, 88, 105, 112, 137
Animal Protein:	82-Crab, crayfish, lobster, prawn, shrimp. 87-Cod, haddock. 88-Ocean catfish. 105-Herring, sardine. 112-Catfish species. 137-Beef (butter, cheese, kefir, milk, veal, yogurt), buffalo, goat, sheep (lamb, mutton).
Vegetables:	2-Mushroom, truffle. 6-Corn, bamboo shoots. 74-Eggplant, sweet pepper, potato, tomato.
Fruit:	34-Avocado. 40a-Apple, crabapple, loquat, pear, quince. 42-Carambola. 46-Acerola. 52-Dried currants, grape, raisin. 61-Pomegranate.
Seeds and Nuts:	22-Hickory nut, pecan, walnut. 62-Brazil nut.
Fats and Oils:	6-Corn oil, rice oil. 22-Walnut oil. 34-Avocado oil. 137-Butter and any fat from above.
Other:	2-Yeast. 6-Barley, cornmeal, corn starch, millet, oats, oat flour, rice, rice flour, rye, rye flour, wheat, wheat flour. 52-Cream of tartar. 74-Potato meal, potato starch.
Sweeteners:	6-Grain syrups: barley, corn, malt, molasses and sorghum. 52-Raisin.
Herbs and Spices:	6-Lemon grass. 34-Bay leaf, cassia, cinnamon. 35-Poppyseed. 73-Applemint, basil, mint, lemon balm, marjoram, oregano, peppermint, rosemary, sage, spearmint, summer savory, thyme, winter savory. 74-Cayenne pepper, chili pepper, paprika, pimiento.
Beverages:	Juice, soup and tea from any of the above. 73-Tea from catnip, chia seed, dittany, horehound, hyssop, pennyroyal. 137-Milk.

SUGGESTED MENUS FOR DAYS 1, 5, 9, ETC.

Breakfast	*Lunch*	*Dinner*
Grape juice or grapes Oatmeal with nut milk Walnuts and/or raisins	Sardines Apples and apple juice Avocado	Tomato juice Raw tomatoes Raw green peppers Beef stew
Grape juice Granola with milk or Oatmeal with butter and milk	Rice wafers or bread Sardines Pecans and/or raisins	Tomato juice Stuffed peppers Avocado, wheat sprouts Popcorn for snack
Apple juice Potato pancakes Applesauce	Baking powder biscuits Whole wheat, sprouted wheat or bat- ter bread Cheese with wheat sprouts Walnuts and dried currants or raisins	Spanish rice, spaghetti or pizza Vegetable salad Grape pie or applesauce cake with milk
Pears and/or pear juice Rice pancakes with pear sauce	Fruit salad with cottage cheese Applesauce cookies with milk	Hamburgers Vegetable salad Wheat balls Milk shake

39

BISCUITS, CRACKERS AND MUFFINS

BAKING POWDER BISCUITS

2 *cups flour*
1 *tablespoon baking powder*
1 *teaspoon sea salt*

⅓ *cup oil of the day*
⅔ *cup milk or water*

Preheat oven to 475°F. Sift together three times all dry ingredients. Combine but do not stir liquids. Add liquid all at once to flour mixture.

Variations:

DROP BISCUIT: Drop onto ungreased cookie sheet. Bake 10–12 minutes.

ROLL BISCUIT: Roll or pat dough to ¼″ or higher. Use unfloured biscuit cutter. Bake 10–12 minutes.

SWEET ROLL: Roll out and sprinkle with raisins, apples or pecans; shape and bake.

POT PIES: Use ¼″ thickness. Filling and dish must be hot—as close to boiling as possible. Bake 12–15 minutes.

RICE WAFERS

½ *cup rice (gritty)*
½ *cup rice polish*
½ *teaspoon baking powder*
½ *teaspoon sea salt*

1 *tablespoon potato starch*
½ *cup pecans, ground*
½ *cup grain syrup*
⅜ *cup oil of the day*

Preheat oven to 425°F. Mix ingredients. Pat batter onto 9″ × 9″ oiled pan. Bake 10–20 minutes.

ROLLED OAT MUFFINS

1 cup rolled oats, ground
¾ cup rice flour
2 tablespoons baking powder
1 teaspoon sea salt
¼ cup butter or beef fat, melted

1 teaspoon cinnamon
⅛ cup grain syrup
  (2 tablespoons)
1⅛ cups water
½ cup raisins

Preheat oven to 425°F. Grind rolled oats in food chopper, using fine cutting blade. Grease muffin tins with oil of the day. Mix dry ingredients thoroughly. Add raisins, water and fat. Then add syrup and mix well. Fill muffin tins about two-thirds full. Bake 20 minutes or until lightly browned. Makes 12 medium-sized muffins.

RYE CRACKERS

1¾ cups rye flour
1 cup rice flour
1½ teaspoon sea salt

1 teaspoon baking soda
½ cup butter or beef fat
1 cup buttermilk

Preheat oven to 375°F. Mix dry ingredients thoroughly. Mix in fat only until mixture is crumbly. Add buttermilk and mix well. Place dough on a well-floured surface. Roll very thin. Cut into strips 3 × 1½ inches. Place with sides touching on baking sheet. Bake 18 minutes or until lightly browned. Makes 75 crackers. Note: Sprinkle top of crackers with coarse salt before baking, if desired.

RYE MUFFINS

1¼ cups rye flour
½ cup rice flour
4 teaspoons baking powder
¼ cup melted butter or beef fat

¾ teaspoon sea salt
⅛ cup grain syrup
1 scant cup water

Preheat oven to 375°F. Mix dry ingredients thoroughly. Add grain syrup, water and fat; mix well. Fill muffin tins (greased with oil of the day) about half full. Bake 25 minutes or until lightly browned. Bakes 12 small muffins.

BREAD RECIPES

HINTS ON MAKING BREAD

Always have kitchen warm when making bread. Avoid drafts. The oven is an excellent place for bread to rise. Turn oven on and set at *warm* for only five minutes before turning off again. Water must be lukewarm before adding yeast. To "punch down" simply beat bread with your fist. This is important, as it helps the fermentation or yeast growth by moving the yeast cells to a new food supply, so that they can grow and multiply. Except for the flour used on hands and beneath bread while kneading, do not add flour after fermentation has begun.

BARLEY BAKING POWDER BREAD

1 cup plus 1 tablespoon whole barley flour	1 teaspoon grain syrup
2 teaspoons melted butter or oil of the day	3 teaspoons baking powder
	¼ teaspoon sea salt
	1 cup water

Preheat oven to 350°F. Sift flour before measuring. Mix dry ingredients. Combine water, oil, syrup and add to dry ingredients, using long strokes. Bake in 4 × 7 × 2″ pan for 25 minutes.

CORN BREAD #1

1 cup cornmeal	1 teaspoon sea salt
¼ cup corn oil	1 teaspoon baking powder
½ cup water	

Preheat oven to 450°F. Mix all ingredients. Pour batter into 9″ × 9″ pan greased with oil of the day. Bake 10–15 minutes.

OATMEAL SHEET BREAD WITH NUTS

1 cup oat flour
1 tablespoon potato starch
1 teaspoon sea salt
⅔ cup water

2 teaspoons baking powder
2 tablespoons oil of the day
⅓ cup nuts (pecans or walnuts)

Preheat oven to 475°F. Mix ingredients. Pat batter onto oiled 9″ × 9″ pan greased with oil of the day. Bake 10–20 minutes.

RAISIN BREAD

1 cup chopped raisins
2 teaspoons baking soda
2 teaspoons baking powder
1 cup potato flour

1 teaspoon sea salt
1½ cups warm water
1 cup butter or corn oil
⅓ cup grain syrup

Preheat oven to 350°F. Let raisins soak in warm water until water cools; add baking soda, butter or oil, syrup, baking powder, potato flour and salt. Bake 45 minutes in loaf pan greased with corn or rice oil.

WHOLE WHEAT BATTER BREAD

1½ cups warm water
2 tablespoons grain syrup
3 tablespoons butter
1⅔ cups unsifted, unbleached flour

1 package yeast
2 teaspoons sea salt
1½ cups unsifted whole wheat flour

Preheat oven to 375°F. Measure warm water and sprinkle yeast on top. Stir until dissolves. Put whole wheat flour in large warm bowl; add yeast, and water, syrup, salt and butter. Beat 2 minutes at medium speed of mixer or 300 strokes by hand. Stir in unbleached flour with wooden spoon. Batter will be quite stiff. Beat until well blended (about 2 minutes). Cover, let rise in warm place free from drafts, about 50 minutes or until double in bulk. Bake 45 to 50 minutes or until bread sounds hollow when tapped on the bottom.

CANDY, DESSERT AND SNACKS
(Also See Pies)

APPLES, BAKED

Cut the tops out of the apples, funnel-shaped; then dig out most of the core with a teaspoon, being careful not to get to the bottom. Place in a baking dish, fill apples with walnuts, and top off with a pinch of mint or cinnamon on each. Surround apples with a cup of water and bake at 350°F. until tender. Eat hot or cold.

APPLES, GLAZED

Pare and core small tart apples. Place in greased baking pan or casserole and sprinkle with 1 part grain syrup mixed with 3 parts boiling water. Bake in moderate oven (350°F.) uncovered for about ½ hour or until tender. Baste syrup over apples 2 or 3 times during cooking for an attractive glaze. Fill centers with raisins and/or pecans.

APPLESAUCE CAKE

½ cup grain syrup
1 cup unsweetened applesauce
½ cup butter
1 teaspoon baking soda
1¾ cups unbleached flour

1 cup raisins
1 cup nuts
1 teaspoon ground cassia
   (optional)

Preheat oven to 375°F. Mix butter and syrup. Add sifted flour, soda and spices, then applesauce. Stir well. Bake in sheet pan until done, 35–40 minutes.

APPLESAUCE COOKIES

¼ cup butter
1¼ cups grain syrup
⅓ cup thick applesauce
1 cup potato starch

¼ teaspoon sea salt
2 teaspoons baking powder
½ cup nuts (pecans or walnuts)

Preheat oven to 350°F. Cream butter and grain syrup. Add applesauce. Mix and sift dry ingredients and stir into mixture. Add nuts. Drop onto cookie sheet. Bake for about 12 minutes.

GARNISHED BREAD SNACKS

Home-made bread sliced rather thin, and buttered. Sprinkle
with spearmint, mint, marjoram and/or cinnamon; toast lightly
under the broiler until golden brown. Eat hot.

GELATIN DESSERT

One package pure gelatin plus 2 cups apple or grape juice.
Soften gelatin in 1 cup of above liquid and dissolve by heating.
Then add rest of liquid. Mold and chill.
   Variation: Add apples and/or pecans.

MOLASSES CRISPS

1¼ cups flour
¾ teaspoon baking soda
¼ cup butter

½ cup molasses or other grain
   syrup

Preheat oven to 375°F. Bring syrup and butter to a boil. Cool
slightly. Add sifted dry ingredients. Chill, roll and cut. Bake
on buttered sheets for 8–10 minutes. Makes 2 dozen.

MOLASSES MOUNDS

4½ cups unbleached wheat flour
1 cup bran
1 teaspoon baking soda
2 teaspoons baking powder

1½ cups molasses
1 cup + 2 tablespoons oil of the
   day
⅓ cup water

Preheat oven to 350°F. Mix dry ingredients in one bowl. Mix
liquid ingredients in another, putting oil in first. Blend
together. Batter should look shiny; if it does not, add more
oil. Roll in balls without pressing down. Place on ungreased
pan and bake 7 minutes exactly.
   Variation: Add 1–2 teaspoons cinnamon.

WHEAT BALLS

1 cup sprouted wheat   2 cups seedless raisins
1 cup brazil nuts or pecans   pinch of sea salt

Grind all ingredients through a food mill, add salt and mix. Make into one-inch balls. Use as a dessert.

    Variation: Two raw apples, grated fine, may be used as well as dried apples or pears.

DAIRY PRODUCTS

BUTTERMILK

Powdered dry skim milk
Commercial buttermilk (unpasteurized)

Make up recipe on box for 1 quart skim milk but use 1 cup less water than called for. Then add 1 cup commercial buttermilk and stir until blended (this gives you a source of preferred bacteria—after the first time, you can use 1 cup of your own as a starter). Add a dash of salt and stir well. Let set at room temperature 24 hours. Stir and use.

COTTAGE CHEESE (LOW FAT)

Make up buttermilk as described in previous recipe and allow to stand 48 hours or until the bottom third of liquid is clear (curds and whey). Do not stir. Gently pour into cloth-lined colander and larger strainer and allow to drain. Use as cottage cheese.

COUNTRY COTTAGE CHEESE

Heat sour milk until the whey (clear liquid) comes to the top. Do not boil! Pour off the whey and put the curd into a cheese cloth bag. Let it drip for six hours without squeezing the bag. Put it into a bowl and chop to desired coarseness. Salt to taste. Add cream if you wish, or work it to the texture of soft putty (paste) adding a little cream and butter as needed.

Mold with hands into pats or balls. Keep in a cool place. Best when fresh.

Variation: Fried Cheese (India-CHANNA): Instead of chopping the curd, cut it into little cubes or slices and fry lightly at moderate heat until golden. Salt and serve. Eat plain or as garnish over vegetables.

MARJORAM MILK

For a soothing cup late at night: a sprig of sweet marjoram in a cup of warm milk. Sweeten to taste (optional).

MILKSHAKE

Chill dried skim milk in freezer compartment; then whip with molasses, cinnamon or mint.

FISH AND MEAT

BASIC MEAT LOAF

1½ pounds ground meat   *1½ teaspoons sea salt*
¼ to ½ cup starch   *½ to 1 cup liquid*

Preheat oven to 325°F. Mix well, form into loaf. Bake 1–1½ hours.

For ground meat use: ground beef, buffalo, goat or lamb.
For starch use: potato meal, riced cooked potato or raw grated potato or corn meal.
For liquid use: meat juice/or gravy, tomato juice, milk or milk substitute.
Season with: ⅛ teaspoon marjoram and ⅛ teaspoon thyme or ¼ teaspoon rosemary and ¼ teaspoon savory. Chopped cooked liver may be mixed into meat.

BEEF STEW

Combine: Cubes of beef with potatoes and green peppers.
Optional: Flavor with bay leaf or herbs from mint family.
Optional: Add ñame, mushrooms and/or tomatoes.

Place in crock pot for 6 to 8 hours.

COUNTRY PIE

1 to 1½ pounds ground beef
1 tablespoon mint, chopped fine
1 teaspoon sea salt

2 tablespoons green pepper,
*   chopped fine*
4 cups or more Spanish rice
*   see page 50*

Preheat oven to 350°F. Combine beef, mint, green pepper
and salt and press into pie dish as for a pie crust. Fill crust
with Spanish rice. Cover with ovenproof lid of reasonable
size. Bake for 25 minutes. Uncover. Bake 10–15 minutes
longer. Serve with grated cheese if desired.

JELLIED VEAL LOAF

1 veal knuckle bone, sawed in
*   half or 2 tablespoons gelatin*
1 pound diced veal
1 bay leaf, or ¼–½ teaspoon other
*   herb (Mint Family, #73)*

bits of red (chopped tomato
*   and/or red sweet pepper)*

Combine and cover with water. Simmer 2 hours. Remove
veal and bone. Chop meat into fine bits. Strain broth and
cook down to make 1 cup. (If using gelatin, add to broth and
stir until dissolved.) Oil loaf pan (sides and bottom) with oil of
the day. Add meat and slice with sharp knife. Veal bones will
make a broth that jells. Other meats must have gelatin added.
Veal has so mild a flavor that it needs extra flavor from herbs
and vegetable juices (instead of water).

MEATBALLS

1 pound ground meat
½ cup rice, raw
2–4 teaspoons finely chopped
  green pepper

1½ teaspoons sea salt
2 tablespoons fine chopped mint,
  if desired

Mix and shape into 8–12 balls. Brown. Add 3½ cups tomatoes. Simmer until done (30–45 minutes), or cook in pressure cooker for 20 minutes.

PIZZA

For the crust: Use one of the recipes recommended under Pies and Crust section for Day 1. Or you can make miniature pizzas by toasting (on both sides) slices of any of the breads or biscuits recommended for Day 1.

Use as a base: thickened spaghetti meat sauce or tomato paste. Cover with layer of cheese. Sprinkle with oregano.
  Variation: Add chopped or sliced mushrooms and/or chopped sautéed green peppers and chopped meat seasoned with cayenne pepper.

SPAGHETTI MEAT SAUCE

3 tablespoons oil of the day
½ cup chopped green peppers
1 pound fresh sliced mushrooms
1½ pounds ground beef
2½ cups pressed drained
  tomatoes

1–2 tablespoons basil, rosemary
  and/or thyme
salt and cayenne pepper to taste
1 bay leaf (optional)

Sauté green peppers and mushrooms. Add meat and sauté until nearly done. Add tomatoes and seasoning and simmer uncovered 20 or 30 minutes. If more liquid is needed add ½ cup hot beef stock or tomato juice.

For a thicker sauce, add ½ cup homemade tomato paste.

Serve over spaghetti, noodles, rice, or wheat or rye sprouts.
  Variation: Serve over steamed potatoes.
  Variation: Add seasoned meatballs and let simmer for 30 minutes.

SPANISH RICE

Brown 1 to 1½ pounds ground meat. Add:

3½ cups tomatoes, raw or cooked	2 cups water
	2 teaspoons sea salt
2 cups raw brown rice	1 green pepper (chopped)

Combine all ingredients in saucepan with tight fitting lid. Bring to boil, then cook on low heat until rice is tender—about 1 hour.

Variation: *Italian flavor:* ½ teaspoon oregano and ¼ teaspoon thyme.
Spicy flavor: ½ teaspoon basil and dash of cayenne pepper.

Use as filling for baked, stuffed green peppers, tomatoes, etc.

Meat roll: using 1 to 1½ pounds ground meat and 1 teaspoon sea salt, roll meat to make a rectangle 12″ × 15″. Spread rice over this to a depth of no more than ½″. Then roll as for jelly roll. Bake as for Country Pie. Or you can make slices and place them cut side up in dish and bake.

Using seasoned ground beef, make thin patties 4″ across. Place a large spoonful Spanish Rice in center of patty and turn up edges as for a tart. Place in covered frying pan and cook at 300°F. until crust is firm and browned.

SPECIAL FEATURE RECIPE: GAME MEAT SAUCE

2 quarts tomato juice or 1 quart whole tomatoes to 1 pound ground meat. (In large quantities, put more meat in proportion to juice.)

Oregano (½ teaspoon per pound of meat up to 1½ teaspoons)
Green pepper to taste

Flake meat. Put all ingredients together and cook over medium heat, until it comes to boil. Simmer about 3½ to 4 hours. Freeze, if desired.

STUFFED PEPPERS

1 quart tomato juice
1 pound chopped meat

3–4 green peppers
dash of sea salt

Preheat oven to 350°F. Roll meat into balls 1″ in diameter and place in covered saucepan filled with tomato juice. Simmer at very low heat for 2 hours or until juice has turned to sauce. Salt to taste. Core green peppers and blanch by parboiling for 2 minutes. Fill green peppers with thickened sauce and meat and bake in covered pan for 15 minutes.

TAMALE PIE

4 ounces meat (goat, lamb, buffalo, beef, veal)
1 teaspoon sea salt
pinch of basil
pinch of oregano

pinch of thyme
dash of chili or cayenne pepper
1 pint tomatoes
½ cup corn

Cook meat with seasonings. Add tomatoes and corn to meat mixture and simmer until done.

PANCAKES, GRANOLA AND WAFFLES

GRANOLA

3 quarts oats
1 cup oat flour
1 cup water

⅓ cup walnut oil
2 cups walnuts

Mix oats, flour and nuts. Add combined oil and water. Stir well until everything is thoroughly coated. Use more water if needed or more oil if desired. Mixture should be a little moist. Spread evenly on cookie sheets. Bake for 30–40 minutes at 250°F. Let cool on sheets. Store in ½ gallon or gallon jars.

Variation #1: Use corn oil and pecans.
Variation #2: Sweeten with raisins and/or dried apples and pears.
Variation #3: Serve with milk, cream, pecan nut milk and/or sprouted rye seed.

OAT WAFFLES

2¼ cups water
½ teaspoon sea salt
1½ cups rolled oats
1 tablespoon oil (walnut, corn or rice)

Optional: ½ cup walnuts or pecans

Combine ingredients in blender. Blend until light and foamy. Let batter stand for about 10 minutes until it thickens. Just before pouring on waffle iron, blend quickly again. Bake 10–15 minutes.

Note: These take longer to bake than regular waffles. Because they stick, do not try to peek for at least 8 minutes. If they do stick, wait; do not try to open or top and bottom will separate. Ingredients may be combined and allowed to soak for 30 minutes or overnight in refrigerator and then beaten. Vigorous beating is required. Chilling will aid in forming steam to promote rising action.

POTATO PANCAKES

4 large potatoes   *3 tablespoons potato meal*

Peel and grate potatoes and combine with potato meal. On very low heat with oil of the day oil pan and spoon mixture into pan. Brown and turn over. Serve alone or with apple or pear sauce.

Variation: Place in oiled cake dish and bake in oven at very low heat until brown and cooked through.

RICE PANCAKES

2 cups rice polish   *½ teaspoon baking soda*
2 tablespoons syrup of the day   *½ teaspoon sea salt*
3 tablespoons rice bran oil
½ cup dried skim milk (water
  may be substituted)

Add spring water for proper consistency. Bake on griddle greased with corn or rice bran oil. Serve with applesauce.

PIES AND CRUSTS

BARLEY FLOUR PIE CRUST

1½ cups whole barley flour   *4 tablespoons butter*
½ teaspoon sea salt
3 or 4 tablespoons water (ice
  cold)

Preheat oven to 400°F. Sift flour before measuring. Add salt and stir in butter. Gradually add water. Pie crust made from flour other than wheat is hard to handle so do not expect this to roll out as ordinary pie crust will. Roll it, then lift it into pie dish and pat it into shape. Bake for 15 minutes.

GRAPE PIE FILLING

Boil seedless grapes in a little water to make juice. Put grapes through juicer. In the absence of yeast/mold allergy, use bottled grape juice.

Bring to boil: 1 cup grape juice

Thicken with: 2 tablespoons potato starch
                2 tablespoons water

Sweeten to taste with grain syrup.

NUT PASTRY PIE CRUST

½ cup ground walnuts or pecans   ¾ teaspoon sea salt
½ cup water   1 teaspoon potato starch
1 cup oat flour

Preheat oven to 475°F. Mix in combined ingredients. Press into pan. Bake 3–5 minutes. Fill with pie filling and continue baking.

GROUND OATS PIE CRUST

2 cups ground organic oat flakes   6 tablespoons oil of the day
   (in blender, not too fine)   2 tablespoons water
¼ teaspoon sea salt

Preheat oven to 425°F. Toss all ingredients together and press into 9″ glass pie pan (greased with same oil that is used in crust). Bake until lightly browned. Cool completely and fill with pie filling of choice.

OIL PIE CRUST

2 cups sifted unbleached flour 1½ teaspoons sea salt
½ cup oil of the day ¼ cup cold water or milk

Preheat oven to 475°F. Do not mix. Add all at once to flour. Stir lightly until blended. Roll. It is easier to press bottom into pie pan and to pat top flat on a cutting board. Prick both top and bottom well with fork. Bake at 425°F. for 40 minutes. For shell of tart shells, bake for 10 minutes.

SHOO-FLY PIE

Crumbs: 1 cup flour
¼ cup oil of the day
Blend together with pastry blender:
Liquid: ½ cup unsulphured molasses
¼ cup boiling water
Mix and add: ½ teaspoon baking soda dissolved in ½ teaspoon
apple cider vinegar

Stir until foamy. Put almost ⅓ of crumbs in 8″ pie pan, then liquid, then remainder of crumbs on top. Bake in 450°F. oven for 10 minutes, or 350°F. for 30 minutes.

SALAD DRESSINGS, GARNISHES AND SAUCES

AVOCADO SALAD DRESSING

1 ripe avocado
4 tablespoons juice (sour grape or tomato)

Cube avocado into blender with juice. Blend at medium speed. Add more juice if necessary to gain consistency of mayonnaise. This is especially good with fish and seafood. Use as a substitute for mayonnaise.

MINCED BASIL AND MARJORAM

Minced basil and marjoram are good in hamburg croquettes.

MINT GARNISH

¼ cup chopped fresh mint   ½ cup apple cider vinegar
1 tablespoon grain syrup   pinch sea salt

Combine and allow to stand for 2 hours before using. Serve with roasts (especially lamb).

MOLASSES BUTTER

2 cups cooked apples   1 cup molasses

Cook well, stirring constantly, untl thick and buttery. Good with pancakes.

TOMATO PASTE

6 large ripe tomatoes   ¾ teaspoon sea salt
2 tablespoons melted butter or   Optional: ½ teaspoon grain
   oil (corn or rice)   syrup (rice or malt, etc.)
¼ teaspoon paprika

Cook all ingredients over low heat stirring constantly (or use double boiler). Cook until they are the consistency of thick paste. Put paste through strainer or blender at low speed.

TOMATO PASTE OR SAUCE (BLENDER)

2 parts tomatoes (fresh, frozen   Sea salt and cayenne pepper to
   or home canned)   taste
1 part green pepper (fresh or   Optional: herb of the day
   frozen)

To use as a paste: Drain excess juice to be used for sauces. Place in blender at slow speed or puree speed. Include core, skin and seeds which add to flavor in cooking.

To use as sauce: Keep the juice.

TOMATO PASTE (JUICER)

Whenever you juice tomatoes and green peppers, save pulp of seeds and skins. Freeze in small packages and use as paste to flavor and thicken tomato sauces.

Also see Fish, Meat and Meat Sauces.

SALADS AND SIDE DISHES

AVOCADO WHEAT OR RYE SPROUT

1 *cubed avocado*   *wheat or rye sprouts*
3 *cups vegetables (green peppers*
   and tomatoes cut in chunks)

Toss avocado and vegetable. No dressing is needed.

Variation: Take 1 ripe tomato and cut almost through to bottom (leaves attached). Set and spread slightly on mound of wheat or rye sprouts. Fill center of tomato with scoop of mashed avocado to which has been added a few drops of vinegar or sour apple juice. Sea salt to taste.
Variation: Substitute green pepper.

FRUIT SALAD

Combine: Chopped apples, pears and grapes.
Add: Pecans or walnuts.
Optional: Apple juice, yogurt or avocado dressing *(See Salad Dressings)*.

GNOCCHI

½ cup melted suet, beef or goat animal fat or butter
2 cups potato (riced or mashed)
½ teaspoon baking powder
1 teaspoon sea salt
½ teaspoon paprika
½ cup potato meal

Preheat oven to 400°F. Beat ingredients together well. Roll into cylinders 1½" in diameter. Chill. Cut into ¼" slices and indent with finger. Place in baking dish (greased with oil of the day), edges overlapping. Cover with meat or tomato sauce.

> Variation: Add herbs from Mint Family (rosemary and marjoram make a good combination).

NEW HAMPSHIRE BANNOCK

1 cup whole white corn meal
2 tablespoons soft butter
½ teaspoon sea salt
boiling water

Preheat oven to 350°F. Combine corn meal and salt. Pour over this enough boiling water to make batter consistency of thick cream. Add butter. Spread thin in large well-greased pan. Bake for about 45 minutes or until crispy brown.

Serve with melted butter, cream, milk or nut milk.

> Variation: Serve with soup.
> Variation: Sweeten to taste with one of the grain syrups.

VEGETABLE SALAD

Combine: Sprouted wheat or rye, raw sweet green or red peppers and tomatoes.

Dressing: Corn or rice oil flavored with mint (or other herb of the day).

Optional: Flavor with poppy seed.

Optional: Add avocado, raw mushrooms and/or bamboo shoots.

Optional: Add diced steamed potatoes, cheese, diced lobster or shrimp.

Variation: Use avocado dressing: See "Salad Dressings and Garnishes."

WALDORF SALAD

Toss lightly together:

2 cups diced apples   *½ cup seedless raisins*
½ cup chopped walnuts

Serve with avocado dressing.

Variation: Add 1 cup seedless grapes.

CHAPTER EIGHT

MENUS AND RECIPES FOR DAYS 2, 6, 10, ETC.

TABLE OF CONTENTS

FOOD CHART FOR DAYS 2, 6, 10 ETC.

Food Families Used:	*4, 9, 13, 14, 16, 17, 18, 19, 24, 26, 28, 31, 32, 40b, 40d, 47, 50, 63, 64, 66, 69, 71, 72, 79, 98, 107, 109, 111, 117, 120, 122, 126.*
Animal Protein:	*98*-Tuna, mackerel. *107*-Whitefish. *109*-Pike. *111*-Carp, chub. *117*-Frogs legs. *120*-Turtle. *122*-Dove, pigeon (squab). *126*-Turkey, turkey eggs.
Vegetables:	*9*-Malanga. *14*-Ñame, yam. *28*-Beet, chard, spinach. *47*-Yuca. *69*-Olive. *79*-Cucumber, pumpkin, squash, zucchini.
Fruit:	*16*-Banana, plantain. *32*-Cherimoya, Custard apple, pawpaw. *40b*-Apricot, cherry, peach, plum. *63*-Guava. *66*-Bearberry, blueberry, cranberry, huckleberry. *79*-Cantaloupe, melon, watermelon.
Seeds and Nuts:	*24*-Chestnut. *26*-Macadamia. *40b*-Almond. *79*-Pumpkin seed.
Oils:	Fats from any of the above. *40b*-Apricot oil, almond oil. *69*-Olive oil.
Other:	*4, 9, 13, 16, 17, 18, 19, 47*-Arrowroot starch, poi, tapioca starch.
Sweeteners:	*50*-Maple syrup.
Herbs and Spices:	*17*-Ginger, turmeric. *40d*-Burnet. *63*-Allspice, clove. *71*-Comfrey. *72*-Lemon verbena.
Beverages:	Juices, soups and teas from any of the above. *31*-Golden Seal. *64*-American Ginseng, Chinese Ginseng. *71*-Comfrey.

SUGGESTED MENUS FOR DAYS 2, 6, 10, ETC.

Breakfast	*Lunch*	*Dinner*
Apricot juice Cherries and almonds	Tuna fish with olives (and oil) Cucumber, steamed squash, cantaloupe	Turkey Spinach and beets Macadamia nuts and/or bananas
Dried stewed fruit (cherries, apricots, peaches and/or prunes) with almonds Bananas	Tuna salad Pumpkin seed crackers Pumpkin seed butter or almond butter Melon	Roast turkey (with chestnut stuffing) Vegetable salad Squash (baked) Banana nut sundae
Pancakes (arrowroot and pumpkin seed) served with dried fruit jam or blueberry butter	Salad (Vegetable, Turkey) Bananas	Steamed whitefish Zucchini (stuffed) Vegetable salad Cherry almond pie or pudding
Cherry arrowroot pudding with bananas Ginseng tea	Fruit salad Pumpkin seed crackers Almond nut butter	Carp or chub almondine Squash pudding Vegetable salad Cucumbers Banana ice cream with almond cookies

BEVERAGES

COMFREY DRINK

15 almonds (soaked overnight in water)

5 teaspoons pumpkin seeds (soaked overnight in water)

16 ounces juice (cherry)

1 banana

Fill blender above blades with unsweetened juice (approximately 8 ounces). Place softened nuts, seeds and banana in juice and liquefy. Pour this mixture into pitcher. Next, take four large handfuls of green leaves (spinach, beet greens, and, most important, *COMFREY*). Liquefy greens in 8 ounces unsweetened juice. Put the two mixtures together. Do not have mixture too thick. Some like to put combined mixture through a strainer.

Variation: If available, juice green leaves in juicer instead of blender; then mixture will not be too thick. Prepare the rest as above.

BISCUITS, CRACKERS AND MUFFINS

PUMPKIN SEED CRACKERS

3 cups pumpkin seed (before grinding)

Grind seed then add:

⅓ cup ground almonds
¾ teaspoon sea salt

3 tablespoons oil (almond)

Preheat oven to 250°F. Add boiling water to make stiff dough. Oil cookie sheet and roll as thin as possible on sheet. (Keep roller wet with water.) Bake for 10 minutes, then increase to 350°F. for 15 minutes.

DESSERTS AND SNACKS

ALMOND COOKIES

3 cups almond meal (or finely
   ground almonds)
3 tablespoons maple syrup
1½ tablespoons almond oil

1 tablespoon cherry juice
   (optional)
1¼ teaspoon ginger (optional)
Boiling water as needed

Preheat oven to 250°F. Combine all ingredients. Add just enough water to hold the ingredients together. Using wet rolling pin, flatten dough on cookie sheet greased with almond oil. Bake until firm enough to cut into squares.

ARROWROOT PUDDING

2 tablespoons arrowroot starch
1 cup juice (apricot, cherry, peach or blueberry)

Add liquid gradually so the starch does not become lumpy. Heat at medium temperature stirring constantly until it thickens.

Cool and add any fruit and/or nuts of the day. Excellent for pie filling with an almond crust.

   Optional: Sweeten to taste with maple syrup.

BANANA BERRY CRUSH

2 bananas
2 cups blueberry juice

1 cup cherries

Freeze fruit. Puree with juice. Serve alone or topped with almonds or macadamia nuts.

BANANA ICE CREAM

2 bananas
1½ cups nut milk (macadamia or almond)

Cherry juice to taste
½ cup maple syrup
2 tablespoons apricot oil

Mix in blender or mash bananas and mix together with electric beater. Freeze, whip again and re-freeze.

BANANA NUT SUNDAE

2 large or 3 small bananas   chopped almonds

Peel and slice bananas and freeze. Partially defrost. Serve with chopped almonds.

Variation: Sweeten to taste with maple syrup.

DRIED FRUIT (STEWED)

3 cups dried fruit (apricot, cherry, peach, prune)

Cover the fruit with boiling water. Soak overnight until tender.

Variation: Serve with chopped almonds or macadamia nuts.

FISH, FOWL AND MEAT

FISH ALMONDINE

1 fish fillet (whitefish, pike or carp)
¼ cup shredded blanched

almonds
4 tablespoons almond oil

Steam fish 5–8 minutes or until it flakes. Sauté almonds in oil and pour over the fish.

ROAST TURKEY

Preheat oven to 350°F. Rub turkey (including the cavity) with ginger as you would with garlic. Liberally brush turkey with a garnish of ground allspice and almond oil.

Line a roaster (uncovered in the beginning) with ¼ inch of water and place turkey on a rack so that water does not touch it. Baste with garnish twice at ½ hour intervals. If more liquid is needed add water. Lower oven to 250°F.; cover roaster and continue to bake about 6 hours or until meat thermometer registers 190°F.

To bring out the natural juices, for the last half hour pour ¾ cup of juice (blueberry, cranberry or cherry) over turkey and baste every ten minutes.

> Variation: After rubbing cavity with ginger, stuff turkey ¾ full. (*See "Chestnut Stuffing" under Salads and Side Dishes.*)

TUNA FISH

See Salads.

TURKEY LEFTOVERS

See Salads, Vegetables.

PANCAKES

ALMOND ARROWROOT PANCAKES

1 cup arrowroot starch	liquid as needed (water or
1 cup almonds	almond nut milk)

Blend dry mixture at low speed adding liquid. Increase speed. Add only enough liquid to reach the right consistency.

> *NOTE:* Because there is no leavening, the pancake will be flatter than usual. Therefore, the batter should

66

be thicker than usual. As you experiment for the right consistency, remember that it is easier to add liquid than dry mixture. To grease griddle, use almond oil or apricot oil.

Variation: Substitute pumpkin seeds for almonds.
Variation: Serve with dried fruit jam, maple syrup or pureed blueberries.

SALAD DRESSINGS, GARNISHES AND SPREADS

BANANA DRESSING

2 bananas
4 tablespoons maple syrup
2 tablespoons apricot juice

8 teaspoons water
dash of sea salt

Bake or steam bananas. Cool, mash and add other ingredients. Beat well with rotary or electric beater.

BLUEBERRY PUREE

4 cups blueberries
liquid as needed (water or blueberry juice)

Puree blueberries in blender using liquid sparingly. Serve with chopped nuts or with pancakes or crackers.

Optional: Sweeten to taste with maple syrup.

DRIED FRUIT JAM

Drain stewed fruit. Puree in blender.

Optional: Sweeten to taste with maple syrup.

OLIVE OIL DRESSING

3 *parts olive oil*
1 *part cucumber juice (more if desired)*

Add juice slowly to olive oil.

Optional: Add finely minced olives or season with ginger,
turmeric or lemon verbena.

SEED (NUT BUTTER)

1 *cup pumpkin seeds*
1 *tablespoon almond oil (more if needed)*

Grind or blend until smooth and store in refrigerator.

Variation: Substitute almonds for pumpkin seeds.

SALADS AND SIDE DISHES

CHESTNUT STUFFING

2½ *cups cooked chestnuts*   3 *tablespoons almond oil*
4 *to 6 cooked yams*   *sea salt to taste (optional)*

Combine riced chestnuts, mashed cooked yams and almond
oil. Use to stuff turkey or as a side dish.

Variation: Sweeten to taste with maple syrup.
Variation: Season with ½ teaspoon ground ginger.

PLANTAIN, SAUTÉED

1 *plantain*   1 *cup oil of the day*

Cut plantain in rounds. Sauté in oil of the day. Either green
or ripe plantain may be used. Green plantain makes a good
biscuit substitute. Ripe plantain is sweet. Serve with meal or
as a dessert.

SALADS: FRUIT COMBINATIONS

1. Apricot, cherry, peach and almonds.
2. Cantaloupe, honey dew, watermelon and pumpkin seeds.
3. Banana, blueberry, guava and macadamia nuts.

Variation: Serve any of the above with banana dressing
(*See Salad Dressings*).

SALAD, TUNA FISH

Combine tuna fish with raw spinach and cucumbers.

Dressing: Olive or almond oil flavored with allspice,
ground clove or ground ginger.
Optional: Add olives.
Optional: Add diced steamed beets or yams.

SALADS: VEGETABLE COMBINATIONS

1. Beet greens, chard, steamed winter squash and pumpkin seeds (*See olive oil dressing*).
2. Raw spinach, cucumbers and chestnuts with almond oil
and allspice.
Variation: Add diced turkey.

SQUASH, BAKED

1 butternut or acorn squash   2 teaspoons maple syrup
2 tablespoons almond oil   (optional)
¼ teaspoon ground ginger
(optional)

Preheat oven to 350°F. Cut squash in half. Remove seeds.
Combine other ingredients and brush on squash. Bake for 20
minutes or until tender.

Variation: Serve with finely chopped chestnuts.
Variation: Stick a whole clove in the end of each half
squash.

SQUASH PUDDING (BUTTERNUT)

Steam and puree equal amounts of butternut squash and pumpkin. Add ground cloves and/or ginger for flavor.

Variation: Substitute mashed steamed plantain or raw bananas for the pumpkin.

ZUCCHINI, STUFFED

6–8 inch sized zucchini   2 tablespoons almond oil
1 cup chopped spinach
¼ cup finely chopped chestnuts
  or pumpkin seeds

Steam zucchini until tender (7–8 minutes). Drain. Cut lengthwise, scoop out and discard seed. Drain again. Sprinkle remaining shell with salt and stuff with spinach and chestnuts. Place stuffed zucchini in shallow baking pan or oven-to-table dish greased with almond oil. Sprinkle each portion with almond oil. Before serving, reheat for about 20 minutes in a 350°F. oven.

CHAPTER NINE

MENUS AND RECIPES FOR DAYS

3,

TABLE OF CONTENTS

7,

FOOD CHART FOR DAYS 3, 7, 11, ETC.

Food Families Used: 1, 7, 8, 10, 23, 27, 33, 39, 40c, 51, 65, 68, 70, 80, 81, 91, 96, 102, 106, 113, 114, 115, 129, 134.

Animal Protein: 81-Abalone, clam, cockle, mussel, oyster, scallop, snail, squid. 91, 96, 102, 106, 113, 114, 115-All bass, all perch, all trout, croaker, grouper, salmon, sauger, walleye. 129-Rabbit. 134-Swine (bacon, ham, pork).

Vegetables: 7-Chinese water chestnut. 65-Carrot, celeriac (celery root), celery, parsley, parsnip. 70-Sweet potato. 80-Artichoke, dandelion, endive, Jerusalem artichoke, lettuce.

Fruit: 8-Date, coconut. 10-Pineapple. 27-Rhubarb. 39-Currant, gooseberry. 40c-Blackberry, raspberry, strawberry. 51-Litchi. 60-Prickly pear. 68-Persimmon.

Seeds and Nuts: 8-Coconut. 23-Filbert (hazelnut). 80-Sunflower seeds.

Fats and Oils: Fats from any of the above. 80-Safflower oil, sunflower oil.

Other: 1-Agar-agar. 27-Buckwheat. 80-Artichoke flour, sunflower seed meal.

Sweeteners: Date sugar.

Herbs and Spices: 1-Kelp (seaweed). 33-Nutmeg. 65-Anise, caraway, celery seed, chervil, coriander, cumin, dill, fennel. 80-Santolina, tansy, tarragon.

Beverages: Juices, soups and teas from any of the above. 80-Tea from boneset, burdock root, chamomile, chicory, goldenrod, yarrow.

SUGGESTED MENUS FOR DAYS 3, 7, 11, ETC.

Breakfast	*Lunch*	*Dinner*
Buckwheat cereal Coconut milk and dates	Salmon Vegetable salad (lettuce, Jerusalem artichokes, endive, sunflower seeds and oil) Sweet potatoes	Pork stew or rabbit stew Raw carrots, celery Filberts and pineapple
Filberts and strawberry pudding made with agar-agar	Sunflower seed wafers Fruit salad	Steamed salmon or baked trout #1 Buckwheat stuffing Date nut balls with pineapple
Buckwheat pancakes #1 with date nut dressing	Salmon Vegetable salad #1 Baked rhubarb	Roast pork Sweet potato with pineapple Filbert berry pie or pudding
Buckwheat/seed pancakes #2 with pureed pineapple	Vegetable salad #2 Steamed scallops Barbecued spareribs or Filbert berry date pie	Baked fish #2 Baked rhubarb with sweet potato Vegetable salad Date cookies

BEVERAGES

COCONUT CREAM, MILK AND SKIM MILK

1 coconut (fresh or frozen)   water as needed (about 3–4
coconut milk from 1   cups)
  coconut

With ice pick, puncture holes in three eyes of the
coconut. Drain coconut milk, strain and refrigerate.

To make it easier to crack coconut shell, place it in oven
for 15 or 20 minutes at 250°F.

Cut coconut into cubes, cover with water (about 3 cups)
and soak overnight in covered jar.

Pour contents of jar into blender. Blend first on low
speed and then on high. Strain liquid to separate it
from shredded coconut. Combine liquid with coconut
milk to make coconut cream.

Return shredded coconut to blender. Cover with more
water, only enough to let blender work. This time
when you strain it you will have coconut skim milk.

    Variation: Use coconut cream as you would regular
                milk. It is good just as a drink by itself or
                seasoned with nutmeg, with sunflower
                seed wafers or date cookies. Serve it on
                buckwheat cereal with strawberries. As a
                special treat serve it with plain fresh
                strawberries.
    Variation: To add a coconut flavor to any recipe
                substitute coconut skim milk for water.
        Note: Check with your produce manager to learn
                the peak of the coconut season when they
                are least expensive. Buy them in quantity,
                freezing the extra coconuts, 1 per pack-

age so you will know how much you are using. Freeze the coconut milk in ice cube trays and store in packages with each frozen coconut.

PIÑA COLADA

1 part coconut cream
1 part pineapple chunks or pineapple juice

Combine in blender.

BISCUITS AND WAFERS

SUNFLOWER SEED WAFER

Blend sunflower seed in blender quite fine. Mix with water moist enough to handle. Make patties about ¼″ thick. Bake on ungreased sheet at moderate temperature until brown. Turn and brown other side.

DESSERTS AND SNACKS

DATE COCONUT COOKIES

1 cup chopped dates
1 cup shredded coconut
½ teaspoon baking soda
⅓ cup artichoke starch

¼ teaspoon salt
spring water as needed
1 teaspoon oil of the day

Preheat oven to 375°F. Cover dates with water, bring to boil and cool. Mix together all dry ingredients and add dates, water and oil of the day. Drop onto greased cookie sheets. Bake until brown (10–12 minutes).

DATE COOKIES

2 cups pitted dates (moist)   *2 cups coconut meal*

Put moist dates in blender or food processor; and grind to a sticky consistency. (Dates that have become too dry will not work.) Shape into balls and roll in the coconut meal. Store in covered container and keep in cool place. You can press whole filberts or chopped chestnuts into tops of balls for added interest and food value.

> Variation: To add moisture to dates, add coconut milk (no more than a teaspoon at a time or it will run rather than stick together).

DATE NUT BALLS

2 parts pitted dates   *1 part filberts*

Put ingredients through food chopper; form into balls and roll in coconut.

DATE PUDDING

1 pound pitted dates, cut fine   *3 tablespoons oil of the day*
1 teaspoon baking soda   *1½ cups artichoke flour*
¾ cup boiling water   *nutmeg to taste (optional)*

Preheat oven to 375°F. Mix dates, soda and boiling water. Stir well and let cool. Mix oil and flour. Stir into date mixture. Add nutmeg. Pour into well-greased baking dish. Bake about 45 minutes. Serve with a coconut pineapple topping.

DATES, STUFFED

Remove pits from dates and stuff with ground sunflower seed. Roll in freshly grated coconut.

> Variation: Stuff with filberts or pineapple chunks.

76

FRUIT PIE FILLING

½ cup soaked dates (pureed)
1¼ cups water
1 tablespoon juice (pineapple,
  blackberry, strawberry or
  raspberry)

⅛ teaspoon sea salt
1 cup pureed berries
2 tablespoons agar-agar flakes
1 cup fresh pineapple

Bring first 5 ingredients to a boil. Add agar-agar flakes; cook 15 minutes. Cool. Add fresh fruit and pour into filbert pie shell. Top with shredded coconut or finely ground filberts.

See Chapter 6 for pie of the day.

FISH, FOWL AND MEAT

FISH, BAKED BATTER

Bass, perch, trout or other fish of the day.

Preheat oven to 400°F. Pour a little water or pineapple juice over fish. Dip in ground filberts, sunflower seed meal or artichoke flour. Bake until fish is flaky (about 10–15 minutes).

Variation: Sauté 3–4 minutes in safflower oil seasoned with dill and/or fennel.

FISH, BAKED

Bass, perch, trout or other fish of the day.

3 pounds fish, dressed
2–3 cups sliced carrots
2–3 cups chopped celery

1 cup water
2 tablespoons minced parsley
1½ teaspoons sea salt

Preheat oven to 350°F. Line pyrex cake dish with vegetables and 1 cup of water. Place fish on top of vegetables. Bake for 25–30 minutes or until fish flakes easily with a fork.

FISH (SALMON)

For any fish as delicate as a salmon steak, place fish on a cake rack, over a broiling pan. Fill bottom of pan with ¼″ water. For an unusual taste season with a little pineapple juice, safflower oil or kelp.

PORK ROAST

1 pork roast   *1 cup pineapple juice*

Preheat oven to 325°F. Pour juice into dish with meat. Bake until tender (about 1 hour).

   Variation: Cook in crock pot for 8–10 hours.

PORK SPARERIBS, "BARBECUED"

12–14 spareribs   *1 cup tarragon*

Partially cook ribs in crock pot (1 hour on high and 3 hours on low). Pour small amount of juice from ribs into pyrex dish. Dip ribs into minced or dried tarragon, and place in pyrex dish in oven for 2 hours (longer if you like it very crisp).

PORK STEW

Season pork with tarragon. Add celery, carrots and parsley.

   Optional: Add parsnips and/or celery root.

Place in crock pot for one hour on high. Turn to low for 6 to 8 hours.

   Variation: Instead of Carrot Family, add Jerusalem artichoke and sweet potato.

RABBITS, DRESSING PROCEDURE

Prepare as you would a chicken.

RABBIT, BILLY CASPER'S FRIED

2 *cleaned young rabbits*   4 *tablespoons tarragon*
1 *cup artichoke flour*   *oil of the day*
salt to taste

Preheat oven to 325°F. Cut rabbits into serving pieces. Place in cellophane bag with seasoned artichoke flour. Close bag and shake vigorously. Pour oil of the day into stainless steel skillet or electric frying pan to ½" depth. Heat oil until sizzling. Cook rabbit in oil, browning on all sides. Finish by roasting crisp 20 minutes or until fork tender.

Variation: Place the floured raw rabbit (seasoned) in a baking dish liberally oiled and bake at 300°F. for 2 hours or until fork tender. This is a healthier procedure.

RABBIT STEW

Combine: Rabbit with carrots, celery and parsley.
Optional: Season with ginger.
Optional: Add Chinese water chestnut, celery root and/or parsnip.

SALAD DRESSINGS, GARNISHES AND SPREADS

DATE NUT SALAD DRESSING

½ *cup boiling water*   ¼ *cup filbert nut butter*
¼ *cup date butter*   ⅛ *teaspoon sea salt*

Pour boiling water over salted "butters." Beat with rotary beater.

RHUBARB, BAKED

2 cups rhubarb, sliced   *boiling water as needed*
½ cup date sugar

Preheat oven to 300°F. Dissolve date sugar in boiling water. Alternate layers of rhubarb and date sugar syrup in a baking dish greased with oil of the day. Bake until rhubarb is red.

Variation: Eat with sweet potatoes or buckwheat pancakes.

SEED/NUT BUTTER

1 cup sunflower seeds   *1 tablespoon safflower oil*

Grind or blend until fine and smooth. Store in refrigerator.

Variation: Substitute filberts for sunflower seeds.

PANCAKES AND CEREALS

BUCKWHEAT CEREAL

½ cup buckwheat   *1 cup water*

Combine and simmer 30 minutes until tender.

BUCKWHEAT PANCAKES #1

¾ cup water   *½ teaspoon sea salt (optional)*
½ cup buckwheat flour

Mix ingredients until full of bubbles. Spoon on hot griddle greased with oil of the day.

BUCKWHEAT SEED CAKES #2

1 cup flour (buckwheat or   *1 cup seed (filbert or sunflower)*
artichoke)   *liquid as needed*

Follow recipe instructions for Example #11 in Chapter 6. Grease grill with safflower or sunflower oil. Serve with pureed strawberries, pineapple or baked rhubarb.

BUCKWHEAT PANCAKES #3

1 cup organic buckwheat flour   *2 tablespoons date sugar*
1 teaspoon sea salt   *(optional)*
1¼ cups water

Stir well, then beat with electric or hand beater until bubbly. Spoon on griddle greased well with oil of the day. Serve with date, coconut, strawberry puree or date/nut salad dressing.

SALADS AND SIDE DISHES

JERUSALEM ARTICHOKES

Prepare by scrubbing and then scraping or peeling thinly. Slice ⅓ to ¼ inches thick and steam about 5–6 minutes.

> Variation: Steam in jackets and peel afterwards.
> Variation: Coat with oil of the day and bake whole at 400°F. for 30 minutes.
> Variation: Sauté.
> Variation: Slice raw for salads.

STUFFING, BUCKWHEAT

Sauté 4 minutes in 3 tablespoons safflower oil:

1 stalk celery   *2 tablespoons parsley*

Add to 2 cups cooked buckwheat. Season with kelp and/or nutmeg.

SWEET POTATO WITH PINEAPPLE

4 large sweet potatoes   *1 pineapple*

Chop and combine steamed sweet potato with pineapple.

SALAD COMBINATIONS (FRUIT)

#1:   Blackberries, strawberries, dates and coconut.
#2:   Pineapple, persimmons, gooseberry and filberts.

SALAD COMBINATIONS (VEGETABLE)

Lettuce, endive, Jerusalem artichoke.

  Optional: Diced, cooked sweet potato.
  Optional: Sunflower seed (roasted or raw).
  Optional: Diced, steamed scallops.

Celery (including yellow and green leaves), carrots and parsley.
(Use sparingly to moderately.)

  Optional: Celeriac (celery root) when available.
  Optional: Diced cooked parsnip.
  Optional: Diced cooked rabbit.

CHAPTER TEN

MENUS AND RECIPES FOR DAYS 4, 8, 12, ETC.

TABLE OF CONTENTS

FOOD CHART FOR DAYS 4, 8, 12, ETC.

Food Families Used: 3, 11, 20, 25, 36, 41, 45, 48, 49, 53, 54, 56, 59, 75, 100, 103, 121, 123, 124, 125, 130.

Animal Protein: 100-Swordfish. 103-Flounder, halibut, sole, turbot. 121-Duck (eggs), goose (eggs). 123-Ruffed grouse (partridge). 124-Chicken (eggs), pheasant, quail. 125-Guinea fowl. 130-Squirrel.

Vegetables: 11-Asparagus, chives, garlic, leek, onion, shallot. 36-Broccoli, Brussels sprouts, cabbage, cauliflower, Chinese cabbage, collards, kale, kohlrabi, mustard greens, radish, rutabaga, turnip, watercress. 41-Alfalfa, all beans, all peas, peanut, soybean. 54-Okra.

Fruit: 25-Fig. 45-Grapefruit, kumquat, lemon, lime, muscat, orange, pummelo, tangelo, tangerine. 48-Mango. 56-Kiwi (Chinese gooseberry). 59-Papaya.

Seeds and Nuts: 41-Peanut, soynut. 48-Cashew nut, pistachio nut. 75-Sesame seed.

Fats and Oils: Fats from any of the above. 41-Peanut oil, soy oil. 75-Sesame oil.

Other: 25-Breadfruit flour. 41-Carob flour, lima bean flour, peanut flour, soy flour. 75-Sesame seed meal, tahini.

Sweeteners: 41-Clover honey, sage honey.

Herbs and Spices: 11-Garlic, chives. 20-Vanilla beans. 36-Horseradish, mustard.

Beverages: Juices, soups and teas from any of the above. 3-Shavegrass. 49-Maté tea. 53-Basswood. 54-Althea root, hibiscus (roselle).

SUGGESTED MENUS FOR DAYS 4, 8, 12, ETC.

Breakfast	Lunch	Dinner
Cashew nuts and figs or mango	Vegetable salad (cabbage, kale, radish, egg or chicken) Sesame seed and oil Papaya	Filet of sole (onions and peanut oil) Asparagus with peanut oil Lima bean and split pea pudding Grapefruit or oranges
Grapefruit Carob pancakes	Peanut crackers Peanut butter Fruit salad	Roast chicken Asparagus Vegetable salad Orange sherbet (with pistachio or cashew nuts)
Oranges Peanut butter waffles	Carob cookies Vegetable salad with chicken or egg	Roast duck Steamed okra Cole slaw Mangoes and cashews
Onion omelet Fruit shake	Egg salad with alfalfa sprouts Peanut crackers Radishes Tangerines or oranges	Lentil soup Baked flounder Vegetable salad Asparagus Protein cake

BISCUITS AND CRACKERS

PEANUT CRACKERS

3 cups peanut flour
1 cup ground sesame seed

¾ teaspoon sea salt
3 tablespoons peanut oil

Preheat oven to 250°F. Combine ingredients. Add enough boiling water to make stiff dough. Grease cookie sheet with peanut oil and roll as thin as possible on sheet. Keep roller wet with water. Bake for 10 minutes, then turn oven to 350°F. for 15 minutes. Cut into squares.

CANDY, DESSERTS AND SNACKS

CANDIED ORANGE PEEL

Peel of 6 medium oranges
1 cup honey

½ cup water

Cut orange peels into sixths. Remove pulp and most of white membrane. Soak overnight in water (weighed down with plate), drain and wash. Cover with cold water and bring to a boil repeating two times (helps remove bitter taste).

Boil 1 cup honey and ½ cup water in a saucepan, add peel and boil until translucent and beginning to candy. Drain in colander and spread on cellophane to dry. Makes about 2 cups.

CAROB ANGEL FOOD CAKE

1 cup carob powder

12 egg whites

Preheat oven to 300°F. Add carob powder to egg whites and beat until very light. Bake from 20 to 30 minutes.

CAROB COOKIES

3 egg whites   ½ cup carob powder

Preheat oven to 300°F. Beat egg whites until very stiff, then fold in carob powder with spatula. Drop on cookie sheet greased with peanut oil and bake 15 minutes. You may add a cashew nut to each cookie before baking if you wish. Honey may be added, if desired, but they are actually sweet with just carob powder.

Variation: Add 1 cup Spanish peanuts to batter.

CAROB PUDDING

3¼ cups water or cashew nut   3 tablespoons carob
  milk   Dash of sea salt
3 tablespoons peanut starch   ¾ cup honey (optional)

Mix to thicken. Stir while cooking. Serve hot or cold.

FIG NUT BALLS

2 parts dried figs
1⅓ parts roasted cashew nuts (or peanuts)

Put 2 parts figs and 1 part nuts through food chopper; form into balls. Crush remaining nuts. Roll the balls in the crushed nuts.

FLOURLESS PIE CRUST

3 egg whites (for a 9″ pan)   Dash of sea salt
2 teaspoons honey

Preheat oven to 300°F. A favorite recipe that is free from all flour is simply egg whites and honey. Make a stiff meringue and form as a crust in the pan. Don't use too much, as it rises. Bake until brown.

FRUIT SHAKE

2 tablespoons soya milk powder   4–6 figs (chopped)
1 pint water

Blend first at low speed; then, at high speed.

NUT COOKIES

1 cup chopped cashew nuts or   ⅓ cup honey
  peanuts   Sea salt
1 egg white, unbeaten

Preheat oven to 325°F. Beat together all ingredients and drop by teaspoon onto well-oiled cookie sheet. Bake 15 minutes. Remove from pan while still warm. Add nut meal if needed for thickening.

NUT SQUARES

2 cups seeds or ground cashew   1 egg white
  nuts   1½ teaspoons sesame seed oil
½ cup honey

Preheat oven to 325°F. Combine over low heat or in top of double boiler. Cool. Shape into balls or roll and cut into squares (between layers of cellophane). Oil hands before shaping balls. Bake on greased cookie sheet for 30–40 minutes. Cool and remove from pan. Add nut meal for body, if needed.

PEANUT BUTTER COOKIES

⅔ cup peanut butter   ½ teaspoon vanilla
½ teaspoon sea salt   2 egg whites, beaten until
2 tablespoons peanut flour   slightly stiff
⅓ cup honey

Preheat oven to 325°F. Combine ingredients in order given. Roll into small balls and place on greased cookie sheet. Crisscross with fork and bake for 12–15 minutes. Yield: approximately 2 dozen.

PROTEIN CAKE

7 eggs, separated
1 teaspoon vanilla
Pinch sea salt

½ pound nuts ground fine
  (cashew)
⅓ cup honey

Preheat oven to 325°F. Beat egg whites until stiff; blend honey, vanilla and salt with egg yolks. Add nuts and mix well. Fold into whites. Place in ungreased angel food pan and bake 1 hour. Invert and separate.

PROTEIN SNACK #2

1 egg, well beaten
¾ cup peanut flour
¾ cup sesame seed meal

2 tablespoons water
1 tablespoon soybean oil
2 tablespoons soybean flour

Preheat oven to 350°F. Mix, drop on greased cookie sheet, press down with fork. Bake about 15 minutes.

SESAME SEED CANDY

2 cups sesame seed
½ cup sesame oil
2 tablespoons honey

½ teaspoon vanilla
1 tablespoon peanut butter
1 tablespoon carob powder

In blender: 2 cups sesame seeds and ½ cup oil. Start blender with cover on and run it a while. Take cover off and help push seeds down and under. Add 2 tablespoons honey and dash of vanilla; blend until smooth. Divide into three bowls. Add 1 tablespoon peanut butter to one; 1 tablespoon carob to another; leave one plain. Shape.

SHERBET

1 cup orange juice or mashed
  papaya
2 egg whites beaten stiff (may
  be omitted if allergic to eggs)

2 cups water
⅔ cup honey

Boil water and honey for 5 minutes. Cool and add fruit juice and put in freezing tray. When firm, remove and mix with stiffly beaten egg whites, beating mixture until light and frothy with electric mixer.

FISH, FOWL AND MEAT

CHICKEN SOUP (CROCK POT)

1 chicken (quartered)
1 medium onion

3–4 cloves garlic

Place ingredients into crock pot on high for one hour. Reduce to low until chicken is fork tender (about 5 hours). Debone chicken. Put bones back into crock pot and fill the crock pot with boiling water. Cook for 2 to 12 hours (the longer the better for strong soup stock).

Optional: Add 2 tablespoons lemon juice.
Optional: Add ½ teaspoon mustard seeds.

Serve with diced chicken, cooked beans and/or peas.

Variation: Serve with uncooked seed sprouts.

CHICKEN GUMBO SOUP

One 4 to 4½ pound stewing chicken, cut up

Add: *2 cups water, ½ teaspoon sea salt*

Cook until tender, about 2 hours. Remove chicken from bones and cube, skim fat from broth.

Combine and add:

4 cups thinly sliced okra   *½ cup chopped onion*
1 teaspoon honey (optional)   *⅛ teaspoon chives*
2 teaspoons sea salt

Cover and simmer ½ hour or until okra is tender. Serves 8.

SESAME CHICKEN OR GUINEA HEN

Preheat oven to 250°F. Dip chicken into beaten egg. Sprinkle generously with sesame seed meal. (Don't dip into the meal. When sesame meal is wet it doesn't cling to the chicken.) Place in baking dish which has been greased with sesame seed oil. Bake for 3–5 hours, depending on how crisp you like it. If you let it bake long enough, it becomes as crisp as fried chicken.

Variation: When time does not permit the slow process, preheat oven to 350°F. and bake for one hour.

Variation: Liberally coat the chicken first with garlic and then with peanut oil or sesame seed oil. Proceed as above.

ROAST CHICKEN

Rub salt and a bit of chives into a frozen fryer (3 pounds plus). Cook in pressure cooker for 30 minutes or less. Remove with great care so it does not fall apart. Fasten legs together with a bit of string. Salt again and add garlic if desired. Broil until browned nicely—only a few minutes. Thicken broth in pressure cooker for gravy, using peanut flour.

PANCAKES AND WAFFLES

CAROB PANCAKES

3 egg yolks
¼ cup water
3 tablespoons carob powder

1 cup peanut starch minus 3 tablespoons
3 egg whites

Spoon onto greaseless electric fry pan (380°F.). Flip once (5–10 minutes).

> Variation: Grease griddle or fry pan with peanut oil or sesame seed oil.

PEANUT WAFFLES

1 cup peanut flour
3 eggs separated and beaten, whites very stiff
¼ cup water or less (add gradually)

2 tablespoons oil (peanut)
¼ teaspoon sea salt
2 tablespoons honey (optional)

Add flour to beaten yolks, then oil and salt. Stir well and add water very gradually, the amount depending on the humidity. When smooth, fold in beaten whites and bake in thoroughly cleaned waffle iron. This is to remove any wheat flour residue. Peanut oil may be used to grease iron if necessary.

SALAD DRESSINGS, GARNISHES, MAYONNAISE AND SPREADS

FIG NUT SALAD DRESSING

½ cup boiling water
¼ cup fig butter
grate orange or lemon rind

¼ cup cashew butter
⅛ teaspoon sea salt

Pour boiling water over nut butter, fig butter and salt. Beat with rotary beater, blender or food processor. Add grated rind to suit taste. Chill. Delicious on fruit salad, as sandwich filler or served with pancakes.

HONEY SAUCE FOR PUDDINGS

1 cup light honey
2 egg whites

dash of sea salt
1 teaspoon ground vanilla bean

Heat honey. Beat egg whites and salt. Then stir in honey in fine stream, continuing to beat until all honey is added. Flavor with powdered vanilla.

ITALIAN DRESSING

1 clove garlic
1 teaspoon honey (optional)
1 teaspoon mustard

1 tablespoon lemon juice
2 tablespoons oil of the day
chopped chives

Pound garlic until smooth. Add mustard and honey. Stir until smooth; add lemon juice drop by drop and beat well. Add oil gradually and follow with sprinkling of chopped chives.

ORANGE FLAVORING

Blend dried peel of organic orange until it becomes a powder. Use this for flavoring in cakes, cookies, custards, etc.

BLENDER MAYONNAISE

1 egg (room temperature)
¾ teaspoon sea salt
½ teaspoon dry mustard

2 tablespoons lemon juice
1 cup oil of the day (room
   temperature)

Put egg, seasonings, lemon juice and ¼ cup of oil into blender and process at blend speed (high speed in a 3-speed blender). Immediately remove top and pour in remaining oil in a steady stream. Turn off. If oil remains, stir with spoon and blend a few seconds more. Repeat until oil disappears.

If this does not thicken, pour ingredients back into measuring cup or other container, leaving ¼ cup of mixture in blender. Add another egg. Proceed as above, pouring remaining ingredients in a steady stream.

MAYONNAISE #2

2 egg yolks
1 cup oil of the day

1 teaspoon sea salt
1 tablespoon lemon juice

Beat salt into unbeaten egg yolks. Add oil very slowly, drop by drop at first, until dressing becomes thick and shiny. (If it curdles, add another yolk, beating this in slowly also.) After ½ oil has been used, add lemon juice.

PEANUT BUTTER

1 cup shelled peanuts

1 teaspoon peanut oil

Put peanuts and peanut oil in blender. Blend with motor on and off to prevent overheating until you have the consistency you want. You can have anything from chunk style to smooth to sloppy. Keep in refrigerator. If you do not like unroasted peanuts, roast them for 20 minutes at 300°F. in their shells, and cool before making them up.

If you have a food processor, omit peanut oil.

SEED/NUT BUTTER

1 cup sesame seeds
1 tablespoon sesame seed oil

½ teaspoon minced chives or
    ground vanilla bean (optional)

Grind or blend until fine and smooth. Store in refrigerator.

Variation: Substitute cashews for sesame seed.

SESAME CREAM

Blend: 1 cup sesame seeds
         1 cup warm water (blend smooth)
         1 tablespoon honey
         dash powdered vanilla beans

   Optional: You may add figs or mango for a different
               flavor.

SESAME NUT CREAM

1 cup sesame milk
½ cup nut butter

6 dried figs, chopped

Blend well and serve over breakfast fruit, or as a sweet
dressing for salads.

SALADS AND SIDE DISHES

ALFALFA SPROUTS

These should never be cooked. Snack on them as is. Put a
handful with favorite spread. Add to salads, cottage cheese,
soup or stew just before serving. Excellent for sandwiches—in
place of lettuce and a lot cheaper.

COLE SLAW

Shred cabbage. Chop up grapefruit and toss with grapefruit
juice. See also "Slaw Supreme."

LEGUMES

1½ cups of dried beans will serve six. Split peas, lentils, pinto beans and blackeyed peas can be cooked without soaking. Other dried legumes should be soaked. Some double in size, lentils more than double, soybeans increase three times their original size.

To retain nutritive value and develop full natural flavor simmer legumes in the water in which they were soaked. Their flavor is enhanced if salt, onions and herbs are added to the soaking and simmering water.

Soybeans are an excellent substitute for meat since ½ cup provides 10 units of protein and only 105 calories. The protein in other legumes is incomplete and must be supplemented with eggs, fish or fowl.

String beans are different if you stir in a raw egg when nearly done. Salt to taste.

NOODLES, PEANUT

Beat until light:

3 egg yolks   *1 whole egg*

Beat in:

3 tablespoons cold water   *1 teaspoon sea salt*

Stir in and work with hands:

2 cups peanut flour

Divide flour into 3 parts. Roll out each piece as thin as possible on lightly floured board. Place between two towels until dough is partially dried. Roll up dough as for jelly roll. Cut with sharp knife into strips of desired thickness. Shake out strips and allow to dry before using or storing.

OKRA, BOILED

Drop into boiling water. With lid on cook 4–5 minutes. Add sea salt and peanut oil and season with lemon juice.

OKRA, SAUTÉED

Southern style: cut okra into small pieces (about ¼" thick). Roll in beaten egg, then roll in peanut flour. Saute in peanut oil at low heat.

OKRA, STEAMED

Okra is good used in soup or cooked with onions. Steam until tender. Season with 2 tablespoons peanut oil, sea salt and 1 teaspoon chives.

SALAD, FRUIT

Combine: Oranges, grapefruit, muscats.
Optional: Add cashews or sesame seeds.
Optional: Add papaya.
Optional: Sweeten with figs.

SALAD, VEGETABLES

Combine: Raw cabbage, watercress and radish.
Dressing: Sesame cream or peanut oil with chives or mayonnaise.
Optional: Lemon juice.
Optional: Sprouts (alfalfa sprouts are particularly good).
Optional: Sesame seeds.
Optional: Chopped eggs or chopped chives.
Optional: Cold cooked beans or peas.

SLAW SUPREME

| 1 head cabbage | 2 tablespoons lemon juice |
| 1/2 cup mayonnaise | 4 chopped scallions |

Cut cabbage into thinnest shreds possible. Place in large bowl and combine with mayonnaise thinned with lemon juice. Add scallions.

   Variation: Use chives, onions or shallots instead of scallions.

SPLIT PEA OR LENTIL SOUP

| 1–1½ cups lentils or split peas | 1 quart water |
| 1 diced onion | sea salt to taste |

Fill large sauce pan with water. Add lentils (depending upon thickness desired) (or dried peas) and onion. Cook slowly 1–2 hours. Add boiling water when necessary.

SPLIT PEA/LIMA BEAN PUDDING

| 1½ cups split peas | 6 cups water |
| 1 cup dried lima beans | sea salt to taste |

Place lima beans in quart container, cover with water and soak overnight. Drain off water into 4-quart pan, adding enough water to make 6 cups. Bring to boil on high heat. Reduce heat to low and add dried peas and soaked beans. After 1 hour, stir every 10 or 15 minutes.

If necessary, add enough boiling water to keep beans from thickening and burning.

   Variation: Serve in soup or as vegetable. Use liquid as stock.
   Variation: Cook down until water evaporates and serve as pudding. This process requires close attention as pudding thickens.

TOFU

1 quart soybean milk
1½ tablespoons lemon juice mixed with ¼ cup water

Bring soybean milk to boil, cooking until quite thick. Turn off
heat and add mixture of lemon juice and water. Stir and let
set a few minutes until milk curdles. Pour into cheese-cloth.
Tie and hang overnight to let liquid drain into bowl, leaving
tofu inside cheesecloth.

Any tofu not used immediately must be placed in glass jar,
covered with water and stored in refrigerator.

Season with chives and serve on peanut crackers.

Season with horseradish or mustard and serve with alfalfa
sprouts and salad.

APPENDIX A

LIST 1
FOOD FAMILIES (ALPHABETICAL)

A

81	abalone
80	absinthe
41	acacia (gum)
46	acerola
79	acorn squash
1	agar-agar
12	agave
98	albacore
41	alfalfa
1	Algae
63	allspice
40b	almond
11	*Aloe vera*
54	althea root
12	Amaryllis Family
94	amberjack
86	American eel
117	Amphibians
85	anchovy
65	angelica
65	anise
38	annatto
136	antelope
40a	apple
73	apple mint
40b	apricot
47	arrowroot, Brazilian (tapioca)
9	arrowroot (*Colocasia*)
17	arrowroot, East Indian (*Curcuma*)
19	Arrowroot, Family

13	arrowroot, Fiji (*Tacca*)
4	arrowroot, Florida (*Zamia*)
19	arrowroot (*Maranta* starch)
16	arrowroot (*Musa*)
18	arrowroot, Queensland
80	artichoke flour
9	Arum Family
11	asparagus
2	*Aspergillus*
34	avocado

B

2	baker's yeast
6	bamboo shoots
16	banana
16	Banana Family
46	Barbados cherry
6	barley
73	basil
114	bass (black)
113	bass (yellow)
53	basswood
34	bay leaf
41	bean
132	bear
66	bearberry
24	Beech Family
137	beef
28	beet
74	bell pepper
73	bergamot
23	Birch Family

121	birds
38	Bixa Family
114	black bass
40c	blackberry
41	black-eyed peas
21	black pepper
80	black salsify
22	black walnut
66	blueberry
93	bluefish
80	boneset
98	bonito
79	Boston marrow
71	borage
71	Borage Family
40c	boysenberry
137	Bovine Family
6	bran
52	brandy
47	Brazilian arrowroot
62	Brazil nut
25	breadfruit
2	brewer's yeast
36	broccoli
36	brussels sprouts
27	buckwheat
27	Buckwheat Family
6	bulgar
80	burdock root
40	burnet
31	Buttercup Family
79	buttercup squash
101	butterfish
22	butternut
79	butternut squash

C

36	cabbage
55	cacao
60	Cactus Family
70	camote
6	cane sugar
18	Canna Family
79	cantaloupe
37	caper
37	Caper Family
74	*Capsicum*

42	carambola
65	caraway seed
17	cardamom
80	cardoon
135	caribou
41	carob
111	carp
29	Carpetweed Family
1	carrageen
65	carrot
65	Carrot Family
79	casaba melon
79	caserta squash
48	cashew
48	Cashew Family
47	cassava
34	cassia bark
47	castor bean
47	castor oil
88	catfish (ocean)
112	catfish species
73	catnip
36	cauliflower
104	caviar
74	cayenne pepper
65	celeriac
65	celery
80	celtuce
9	ceriman
80	chamomile
52	champagne
28	chard
79	chayote
32	cherimoya
40b	cherry
65	chervil
24	chestnut
73	chia seed
124	chicken
41	chickpea
67	chicle
80	chicory
74	chili pepper
36	Chinese cabbage
56	Chinese gooseberry
14	Chinese potato
79	Chinese preserving melon
7	Chinese water chestnut

O

6	oat
6	oatmeal
88	ocean catfish
102	ocean perch
23	oil of birch
54	okra
69	olive
69	Olive Family
11	onion
128	opossum
45	orange
20	Orchid Family
73	oregano
15	orris root
42	oxalis
42	Oxalis Family
81	oyster
80	oyster plant

P

8	palm cabbage
8	Palm Family
59	papaya
59	Papaya Family
74	paprika
62	paradise nut
65	parsley
65	parsnip
123	partridge
58	Passion Flower Family
58	passion fruit
6	patent flour
79	pattypan squash
32	pawpaw
41	pea
40b	peach
124	peafowl
41	peanut
40a	pear
22	pecan
40a	pectin
75	Pedalium Family
73	pennyroyal
74	pepino

74	pepper, sweet
21	peppercorn
21	Pepper Family
73	peppermint
102	perch (ocean)
113	perch (white)
115	perch (yellow)
79	Persian melon
68	persimmon
124	pheasant
109	pickerel
122	pigeon (squab)
30	pigweed
109	pike
84	pilchard (sardine)
63	*Pimenta*
74	pimiento
10	pineapple
10	Pineapple Family
5	pine nut
21	*Piper*
48	pistachio
103	plaice
16	plantain
40b	plum
9	poi
48	poison ivy
87	pollack
61	pomegranate
61	Pomegranate Family
94	pompano
6	popcorn
35	Poppy Family
35	poppyseed
97	porgy
74	potato
74	Potato Family
82	prawn
79	preserving melon
60	prickly pear
26	Protea Family
40	prune
2	puffball
12	pulque
45	pummelo
79	pumpkin

114	pumpkinseed (sunfish)	80	santolina
30	purslane	67	Sapodilla Family
30	Purslane Family	62	Sapucaya Family
80	pyrethrum	62	sapucaya nut
		84	sardines (pilchard)
	Q	11	sarsaparilla
		34	sassafras
124	quail	115	sauger (perch)
18	Queensland arrowroot	73	savory
26	Queensland nut	39	Saxifrage Family
40	quince	81	scallop
		80	scolymus
	R	80	scorzonera
		91	Sea Bass Family
129	rabbit	27	sea grape
36	radish	84	sea herring
52	raisin	96	sea trout
11	ramp	1	seaweed
36	rape	7	Sedge Family
40	raspberry	41	senna
119	rattlesnake	75	sesame
41	red clover	105	shad
135	reindeer	11	shallot
118	Reptiles	3	shavegrass
27	rhubarb	137	sheep
6	rice	82	shrimp
137	Rocky Mountain sheep	96	silver perch
105	roe	90	silverside
80	romaine	98	skipjack
40	Rose Family	40b	sloe
102	rosefish	108	smelt
40	rosehips	81	snail
54	roselle	51	Soapberry Family
73	rosemary	11	soap plant
45	Rue Family	103	sole
123	ruffed grouse	6	sorghum
36	rutabaga	27	sorrel
6	rye	80	southernwood
		41	soybean
	S	41	soy products
		73	spearmint
80	safflower oil	28	spinach
15	saffron	96	spot
73	sage	96	spotted sea trout
8	sago starch	47	Spurge Family
99	sailfish	79	squash
106	salmon species	81	squid
80	salsify	130	squirrel

Z

LIST 2
FOOD FAMILIES (NUMERICAL)

PLANT

1 Algae
    agar-agar
    carrageen (Irish moss)
    *dulse
    kelp (seaweed)
2 Fungi
    baker's yeast ("Red Star")
    brewer's or nutritional yeast
    mold (in certain cheeses)
    citric acid *(Aspergillus)*
    morel
    mushroom
    puffball
    truffle
3 Horsetail Family
    *shavegrass (horsetail)
4 Cycad Family
    Florida arrowroot *(Zamia)*
5 Conifer Family
    *juniper (gin)
    pine nut (piñon, pinyon)
6 Grass (Grain) Family
    bamboo shoots
    barley
      malt
      maltose
    corn (mature)
      corn meal
      corn oil
      cornstarch
      corn sugar
      corn syrup
      hominy grits
      popcorn
    lemon grass
      citronella
    millet
    oat
      oatmeal
    rice
      rice flour
    rye
    sorghum grain
      syrup
    sugar cane
      cane sugar
      molasses
      raw sugar
    sweet corn
    triticale
    wheat
      bran
      bulgur
      flour
        gluten
        graham
        patent
        whole wheat
      wheat germ
    wild rice

* One or more plant parts (leaf, root, seed, etc.) used as a beverage.

7 Sedge Family
    Chinese water chestnut
    chufa (groundnut)
8 Palm Family
    coconut
        coconut meal
        coconut oil
    date
        date sugar
    palm cabbage
    sago starch *(Metroxylon)*
9 Arum Family
    ceriman *(Monstera)*
    dasheen *(Colocasia)*
        arrowroot
    taro *(Colocasia)* arrowroot
      poi
    malanga *(Xanthosoma)*
    yautia *(Xanthosoma)*
10 Pineapple Family
    pineapple
11 Lily Family
    Aloe vera
    asparagus
    chives
    garlic
    leek
    onion
    ramp
   *sarsaparilla
    shallot
    yucca (soap plant)
12 Amaryllis Family
    agave
        mescal, pulque and tequila
13 Tacca Family
    Fiji arrowroot *(Tacca)*
14 Yam Family
    Chinese potato (yam)
    ñame (yampi)
15 Iris Family
    orris root (scent)
    saffron (Crocus)
16 Banana Family
    arrowroot (Musa)
    banana
    plantain

17 Ginger Family
    cardamom
    East Indian arrowroot
        (Curcuma)
    ginger
    turmeric
18 Canna Family
    Queensland arrowroot
19 Arrowroot Family
    arrowroot *(Maranta* starch)
20 Orchid Family
    vanilla
21 Pepper Family
    peppercorn *(Piper)*
        black pepper
        white pepper
22 Walnut Family
    black walnut
    butternut
    English walnut
    heartnut
    hickory nut
    pecan
23 Birch Family
    filbert (hazelnut)
    oil of birch (wintergreen)
        (some wintergreen flavor
        is methyl salicylate)
24 Beech Family
    chestnut
    chinquapin
25 Mulberry Family
    breadfruit
    fig
   *hop
    mulberry
26 Protea Family
    macadamia (Queensland nut)
27 Buckwheat Family
    buckwheat
    garden sorrel
    rhubarb
    sea grape
28 Goosefoot Family
    beet
    chard
    lamb's-quarters
    spinach

sugar beet
tampala
29 Carpetweed Family
New Zealand spinach
30 Purslane Family
pigweed (purslane)
31 Buttercup Family
*golden seal
32 Custard-Apple Family
Annona species
cherimoya
custard-apple
papaw (pawpaw)
33 Nutmeg Family
nutmeg
mace
34 Laurel Family
avocado
bay leaf
cassia bark
cinnamon
*sassafras
filé (powdered leaves)
35 Poppy Family
poppyseed
36 Mustard Family
broccoli
brussell sprouts
cabbage
cardoon
cauliflower
Chinese cabbage
collards
colza shoots
couve tronchuda
curly cress
horseradish
kale
kohlrabi
mustard greens
mustard seed
radish
rape
rutabaga (swede)
turnip
upland cress
watercress

37 Caper Family
caper
38 Bixa Family
annatto (natural yellow dye)
39 Saxifrage Family
currant
gooseberry
40 Rose Family
a. pomes
apple
cider
vinegar
pectin
crabapple
loquat
pear
quince
*rosehips
b. stone fruits
almond
apricot
cherry
peach (nectarine)
plum (prune)
sloe
c. berries
blackberry
boysenberry
dewberry
loganberry
longberry
youngberry
*raspberry (leaf)
black raspberry
red raspberry
purple raspberry
*strawberry (leaf)
wineberry
d. herb
burnet (cucumber
flavor)
41 Legume Family
*alfalfa (sprouts)
beans
fava
lima
mung (sprouts)
navy

string (kidney)
black-eye pea (cowpea)
*carob
  carob syrup
chickpea (garbanzo)
*fenugreek
gum acacia
gum tragacanth
jicama
kudzu
lentil
*licorice
pea
peanut
  peanut oil
*red clover
*senna
soybean
  lecithin
  soy flour
  soy grits
  soy milk
  soy oil
tamarind
tonka bean
  coumarin
42 Oxalis Family
carambola
oxalis
43 Nasturtium Family
nasturtium
44 Flax Family
*flaxseed
45 Rue (Citrus) Family
citron
grapefruit
kumquat
lemon
lime
murcot
orange
pummelo
tangelo
tangerine
46 Malpighia Family
acerola (Barbados cherry)
47 Spurge Family
cassava or yuca (*Manihot*)

cassava meal
tapioca (Brazilian
    arrowroot)
castor bean
castor oil
48 Cashew Family
cashew
mango
pistachio
poison ivy
poison oak
poison sumac
49 Holly Family
maté (yerba maté)
50 Maple Family
maple sugar
maple syrup
51 Soapberry Family
litchi (lychee)
52 Grape Family
grape
  brandy
  champagne
  cream of tartar
  dried "currant"
  raisin
  wine
  wine vinegar
muscadine
53 Linden Family
*basswood (linden)
54 Mallow Family
*althea root
cottonseed oil
*hibiscus (roselle)
okra
55 Sterculia Family
*chocolate (cacao)
*cocoa
  cocoa butter
cola nut
56 Dillenia Family
Chinese gooseberry (kiwi)
57 Tea Family
*tea
58 Passion Flower Family
granadilla (passion fruit)

59 Papaya Family
    papaya
60 Cactus Family
    prickly pear
61 Pomegranate Family
    pomegranate
    grenadine
62 Sapucaya Family
    Brazil nut
    sapucaya nut (paradise nut)
63 Myrtle Family
    allspice *(Pimenta)*
    clove
    *eucalyptus
    guava
64 Ginseng Family
    *American ginseng
    *Chinese ginseng
65 Carrot Family
    angelica
    anise
    caraway
    carrot
      carrot syrup
    celeriac (celery root)
    celery
     *seed and leaf
    chervil
    coriander
    cumin
    dill
      dill seed
    *fennel
      finocchio
        Florence fennel
    *gotu kola
    *lovage
    *parsley
    parsnip
    sweet cicely
66 Heath Family
    *bearberry
    *blueberry
    cranberry
    *huckleberry
67 Sapodilla Family
    chicle (chewing gum)

68 Ebony Family
    American persimmon
    kaki (Japanese persimmon)
69 Olive Family
    olive (green or ripe)
    olive oil
70 Morning-Glory Family
    camote
    sweet potato
71 Borage Family (Herbs)
    borage
    *comfrey (leaf and root)
72 Verbena Family
    *lemon verbena
73 Mint Family (Herbs)
    apple mint
    basil
    bergamot
    *catnip
    *chia seed
    clary
    *dittany
    *horehound
    *hyssop
    lavender
    *lemon balm
    marjoram
    oregano
    *pennyroyal
    *peppermint
    rosemary
    sage
    *spearmint
    summer savory
    thyme
    winter savory
74 Potato Family
    eggplant
    ground cherry
    pepino (melon pear)
    pepper *(Capsicum)*
      bell, sweet
      cayenne
      chili
      paprika
      pimiento
    potato

tobacco
tomatillo
tomato
tree tomato
75 Pedalium Family
  sesame seed
    sesame oil
    tahini
76 Madder Family
  *coffee
  woodruff
77 Honeysuckle Family
  elderberry
    elderberry flowers
78 Valerian Family
  corn salad (fetticus)
79 Gourd Family
  chayote
  Chinese preserving melon
  cucumber
  gherkin
  loofah (*Luffa*) (vegetable
    sponge)
  muskmelons
    cantaloupe
    casaba
    crenshaw
    honeydew
    Persian melon
  pumpkin
    pumpkin seed and meal
  squashes
    acorn
    buttercup
    butternut
    Boston marrow
    caserta
    cocozelle
    crookneck and straightneck
    cushaw
    golden nugget
    Hubbard varieties
    pattypan
    turban
    vegetable spaghetti
    zucchini
  watermelon

80 Composite Family
  *boneset
  *burdock root
  cardoon
  chamomile
  *chicory
  coltsfoot
  costmary
  dandelion
  endive
  escarole
  globe artichoke
  *goldenrod
  Jerusalem artichoke
    artichoke flour
  lettuce
    celtuce
  pyrethrum
  romaine
  safflower oil
  salsify (oyster plant)
  santolina (herb)
  scolymus (Spanish oyster
    plant)
  scorzonera (black salsify)
  southernwood
  sunflower
    sunflower seed (meal and
      oil)
  tansy (herb)
  tarragon (herb)
  witloof chicory
    (French endive)
  wormwood (absinthe)
  *yarrow

ANIMAL

81 *Mollusks*
  Gastropods
    abalone
    snail
  Cephalopod
    squid
  Pelecypods
    clam
    cockle
    mussel

oyster
scallop
82 *Crustaceans*
   crab
   crayfish
   lobster
   prawn
   shrimp
83 *Fishes (saltwater)*
84 Herring Family
   menhaden
   pilchard (sardine)
   sea herring
85 Anchovy Family
   anchovy
86 Eel Family
   American eel
87 Codfish Family
   cod (scrod)
   cusk
   haddock
   hake
   pollack
88 Sea Catfish Family
   ocean catfish
89 Mullet Family
   mullet
90 Silverside Family
   silverside (whitebait)
91 Sea Bass Family
   grouper
   sea bass
92 Tilefish Family
   tilefish
93 Bluefish Family
   bluefish
94 Jack Family
   amberjack
   pompano
   yellow jack
95 Dolphin Family
   dolphin
96 Croaker Family
   croaker
   drum
   sea trout

silver perch
spot
weakfish (spotted sea trout)
97 Porgy Family
   northern scup (porgy)
98 Mackerel Family
   albacore
   bonito
   mackerel
   skipjack
   tuna
99 Marlin Family
   marlin
   sailfish
100 Swordfish Family
   swordfish
101 Harvestfish Family
   butterfish
   harvestfish
102 Scorpionfish Family
   rosefish (ocean perch)
103 Flounder Family
   dab
   flounder
   halibut
   plaice
   sole
   turbot
104 *Fishes (freshwater)*
104 Sturgeon Family
   sturgeon (caviar)
105 Herring Family
   shad (roe)
106 Salmon Family
   salmon species
   trout species
107 Whitefish Family
   whitefish
108 Smelt Family
   smelt
109 Pike Family
   muskellunge
   pickerel
   pike
110 Sucker Family
   buffalofish
   sucker

111 Minnow Family	126 Turkey Family
carp	turkey
chub	eggs
112 Catfish Family	127 *Mammals*
catfish species	128 Opossum Family
113 Bass Family	opposum
white perch	129 Hare Family
yellow bass	rabbit
114 Sunfish Family	130 Squirrel Family
black bass species	squirrel
sunfish species	131 Whale Family
pumpkinseed	whale
crappie	132 Bear Family
115 Perch Family	bear
sauger	133 Horse Family
walleye	horse
yellow perch	134 Swine Family
116 Croaker Family	hog (pork)
freshwater drum	bacon
117 *Amphibians*	ham
117 Frog Family	lard
frog (frogs legs)	pork gelatin
118 Reptiles	sausage
119 Snake Family	scrapple
rattlesnake	135 Deer Family
120 Turtle Family	caribou
terrapin	deer (venison)
turtle species	elk
121 *Birds*	moose
121 Duck Family	reindeer
duck	136 Pronghorn Family
eggs	antelope
goose	137 Bovine Family
eggs	beef cattle
122 Dove Family	beef
dove	beef by-products
pigeon (squab)	gelatin
123 Grouse Family	oleomargarine
ruffed grouse (partridge)	rennin (rennet)
124 Pheasant Family	sausage casings
chicken	suet
eggs	milk products
peafowl	butter
pheasant	cheese
quail	ice cream
125 Guinea Fowl Family	lactose
guinea fowl	spray dried milk
eggs	yogurt

veal
buffalo (bison)
goat (kid)
  cheese
  ice cream

milk
sheep (domestic)
  lamb
  mutton
  Rocky Mountain Sheep

APPENDIX B:

DAILY FOOD CHARTS

FOOD CHART FOR DAYS 1, 5, 9, ETC.

Food Families Used: 2, 6, 22, 34, 35, 40a, 42, 46, 52, 61, 62, 73, 74, 82, 87, 88, 105, 112, 137

Animal Protein: 82-Crab, crayfish, lobster, prawn, shrimp. 87-Cod, haddock. 88-Ocean catfish. 105-Herring, sardine. 112-Catfish species. 137-Beef (butter, cheese, kefir, milk, veal, yogurt), buffalo, goat, sheep (lamb, mutton).

Vegetables: 2-Mushroom, truffle. 6-Corn, bamboo shoots. 74-Eggplant, sweet pepper, potato, tomato.

Fruit: 34-Avocado. 40a-Apple, crabapple, loquat, pear, quince. 42-Carambola. 46-Acerola. 52-Dried currants, grape, raisin. 61-Pomegranate.

Seeds and Nuts: 22-Hickory nut, pecan, walnut. 62-Brazil nut.

Fats and Oils: 6-Corn oil, rice oil. 22-Walnut oil. 34-Avocado oil. 137-Butter and any fat from above.

Other: 2-Yeast. 6-Barley, cornmeal, corn starch, millet, oats, oat flour, rice, rice flour, rye, rye flour, wheat, wheat flour. 52-Cream of tartar. 74-Potato meal, potato starch.

Sweeteners: 6-Grain syrups: barley, corn, malt, molasses and sorghum. 52-Raisin.

Herbs and Spices: 6-Lemon grass. 34-Bay leaf, cassia, cinnamon. 35-Poppyseed. 73-Applemint, basil, mint, lemon balm, marjoram, oregano, peppermint, rosemary, sage, spearmint, summer savory, thyme, winter savory. 74-Cayenne pepper, chili pepper, paprika, pimiento.

Beverages: Juice, soup and tea from any of the above. 73-Tea from catnip, chia seed, dittany, horehound, hyssop, pennyroyal. 137-Milk.

118

FOOD CHART FOR DAYS 2, 6, 10, ETC.

Food Families Used: 4, 9, 13, 14, 16, 17, 18, 19, 24, 26, 28, 31, 32, 40b, 40d, 47, 50, 63, 64, 66, 69, 71, 72, 79, 98, 107, 109, 111, 117, 120, 122, 126.

Animal Protein: 98-Tuna, mackerel. 107-Whitefish. 109-Pike. 111-Carp, chub. 117-Frogs legs. 120-Turtle. 122-Dove, pigeon (squab). 126-Turkey, turkey eggs.

Vegetables: 9-Malanga. 14-Name, yam. 28-Beet, chard, spinach. 47-Yuca. 69-Olive. 79-Cucumber, pumpkin, squash, zucchini.

Fruit: 16-Banana, plantain. 32-Cherimoya, custardapple, pawpaw. 40b-Apricot, cherry, peach, plum. 63-Guava. 66-Bearberry, blueberry, cranberry, huckleberry. 79-Cantaloupe, melon, watermelon.

Seeds and Nuts: 24-Chestnut. 26-Macadamia. 40b-Almond. 79-Pumpkin seed.

Oils: Fats from any of the above. 40b-Apricot oil, almond oil. 69-Olive oil.

Other: 4, 9, 13, 16, 17, 18, 19, 47-Arrowroot starch, poi, tapioca starch.

Sweeteners: 50-Maple syrup.

Herbs and Spices: 17-Ginger, turmeric. 40d-Burnet. 63-Allspice, clove. 71-Comfrey. 72-Lemon verbena.

Beverages: Juices, soups and teas from any of the above. 31-Golden Seal. 64-American Ginseng, Chinese Ginseng. 71-Comfrey.

FOOD CHART FOR DAYS 3, 7, 11, ETC.

Food Families Used: 1, 7, 8, 10, 23, 27, 33, 39, 40c, 51, 60, 65, 68, 70, 80, 81, 91, 96, 102, 106, 113, 114, 115, 129, 134.

Animal Protein: 81-Abalone, clam, cockle, mussel, oyster, scallop, snail, squid. 91, 96, 102, 106, 113, 114, 115-All bass, all perch, all trout, croaker, grouper, salmon, sauger, walleye. 129-Rabbit. 134-Swine (bacon, ham, pork).

Vegetables: 7-Chinese water chestnut. 65-Carrot, celeriac (celery root), celery, parsley, parsnip. 70-Camote, sweet potato. 80-Artichoke, dandelion, endive, Jerusalem artichoke, lettuce.

Fruit: 8-Date, coconut. 10-Pineapple. 27-Rhubarb. 39-Currant, gooseberry. 40c-Blackberry, raspberry, strawberry. 51-Litchi. 60-Pricklypear. 68-Persimmon.

Seeds and Nuts: 8-Coconut. 23-Filbert (hazelnut). 80-Sunflower seeds.

Fats and Oils: Fats from any of the above. 80-Safflower oil, sunflower oil.

Other: 1-Agar agar. 27-Buckwheat. 80-Artichoke flour, sunflower seed meal.

Sweeteners: Date sugar.

Herbs and Spices: 1-Kelp (seaweed). 33-Nutmeg. 65-Anise, caraway, celery seed, chervil, coriander, cumin, dill, fennel. 80-Santolina, tansy, tarragon.

Beverages: Juices, soups and teas from any of the above. 80-Tea from boneset, burdock root, chamomile, chicory, goldenrod, yarrow.

FOOD CHART FOR DAYS 4, 8, 12, ETC.

Food Families Used: 3, 11, 20, 25, 36, 41, 45, 48, 49, 53, 54, 56, 59, 75, 100, 103, 121, 123, 124, 125, 130.

Animal Protein: 100-Swordfish. 103-Flounder, halibut, sole, turbot. 121-Duck (eggs), goose (eggs). 123-Ruffed grouse (partridge). 124-Chicken (eggs), pheasant, quail. 125-Guinea fowl. 130-Squirrel.

Vegetables: 11-Asparagus, chives, garlic, leek, onion, shallot. 36-Broccoli, Brussels sprouts, cabbage, cauliflower, Chinese cabbage, collards, kale, kohlrabi, mustard greens, radish, rutabaga, turnip, watercress. 41-Alfalfa, all beans, all peas, peanut, soybean. 54-Okra.

Fruit: 25-Fig. 45-Grapefruit, kumquat, lemon, lime, muscat, orange, pummelo, tangelo, tangerine. 48-Mango. 56-Kiwi (Chinese gooseberry). 59-Papaya.

Seeds and Nuts: 41-Peanut, soynut. 48-Cashew nut, pistachio nut. 75-Sesame seed.

Fats and Oils: Fats from any of the above. 41-Peanut oil, soy oil. 75-Sesame oil.

Other: 25-Breadfruit flour. 41-Carob flour, lima bean flour, peanut flour, soy flour. 75-Sesame seed meal, tahini.

Sweeteners: 41-Clover honey, sage honey.

Herbs and Spices: 11-Garlic, chives. 20-Vanilla beans. 36-Horseradish, mustard.

Beverages: Juices, soups and teas from any of the above. 3-Shavegrass. 49-Maté tea. 53-Basswood. 54-Althea root, hibiscus (roselle).

APPENDIX C

SOURCES OF FURTHER INFORMATION

Write for information.

Human Ecology Action League (H.E.A.L.)
P.O. Box 1369
Evanston, Illinois 60204

A national non-profit organization formed "to focus the energies, activities and attention of all people vitally interested in good 'Human Ecology' and its reverse—'Ecologic Illness.'"

Human Ecology Research Foundation
505 North Lake Drive
Suite 6506
Chicago, Illinois 60611

Human Ecology Research Foundation of the Southwest
12110 Webbs Chapel Road
Suite E305
Dallas, Texas 75234

Society for Clinical Ecology
Del Stigler, M.D., Secretary
2005 Franklin, Suite 490
Denver, Colorado 80205

An organization which can provide names of clinical ecologists in various parts of the United States and abroad.

APPENDIX D

SUGGESTED READING

Crook, William G. 1975. *Can Your Child Read? Is He Hyperactive?* Jackson, Tennessee.: Pedi Center Press.

Crook, William G. 1978. *Tracking Down Hidden Food Allergies.* Jackson, Tennessee.: Professional Books.

Golos, Natalie and Golbitz, Frances Golos with Leighton, Frances Spatz. 1979. *Coping With Your Allergies.* New York: Simon & Schuster.

Hunter, Beatrice Trum. 1971. *Consumer Beware!* New York: Simon & Schuster.

Mackerness, Richard. 1976. *Eating Dangerously: The Hazards of Hidden Allergies.* New York and London: Harcourt Brace Jovanovich.

Randolph, Theron G. and Moss, Ralph W. 1980. *An Alternative Approach to Allergies.* New York: Harper and Row.

Randolph, Theron G. 1962 (sixth printing, 1978). *Human Ecology and Susceptibility to the Chemical Environment.* Springfield, Illinois: Charles C. Thomas.

Rapp, Doris J. 1979. *Allergies and the Hyperactive Child.* New York: Cornerstone Library, Inc.

Rapp, Doris J. 1980. *Allergies and Your Family.* New York: Sterling Publishing Co., Inc.

APPENDIX E

SOURCE FOR UNUSUAL FOODS

Bread everyday on a rotation diet? For people with extreme food sensitivities or for those who just wish to have greater variety, I have finally found a solution. A very inventive mother, Karen Slimak has learned to use exotic foods for her allergic children; she makes and sells flours, pastas and baking powder from different South American tubers. Because the equipment and foods are costly and the work time consuming, the prices are necessarily high. However it gives you an opportunity, without breaking your rotation, to have bread everyday without using grains, eggs, milk or yeast.

Among the products she has developed are baking powders, flours and pasta (fettucine, lasagne, macaroni, noodles and spaghetti) all made from ñame, malanga, cassava, or camote (the South American white sweet potato). She also sells jams made from carambola, cherimoya, custard apple, guava, papaya or prickly pear with nothing added. If none of the above meets your requirements, Karen will welcome a discussion about alternative substitutes. She will also prepare nut butters not available in stores.

The baking powder is made from baking soda, calcium phosphate and her homemade flour of your choice. Before you order the baking powders or flours, I suggest that you test the vegetable tubers from which these are made.

For further information, send a self-addressed envelope to Karen Slimak, 9207 Shotgun Court, Springfield, VA 22153. Phone (703) 644-0991. Karen will include recipes for breads, cookies, pancakes and pastas. She will also send an instruction sheet indicating how to fit her products into our rotation plan.

Natalie Golos

NOTES

1. Natalie Golos and Frances Golos Golbitz. 1979. *Coping With Your Allergies* New York: Simon & Schuster.

2. Theron G. Randolph, M.D. and Ralph W. Moss, Ph.D. 1980. *An Alternative Approach to Allergies* New York: Lippincott and Crowell.

3. Human Ecology Action League. See Appendix C.

4. Doris J. Rapp, M.D. 1979. *Allergies and the Hyperactive Child* New York: Cornerstone Library, Inc.

5. Doris J. Rapp, M. D. 1980. *Allergies and Your Family.* New York: Sterling Publishing Co., Inc.

INDEX

127

Fruit combinations in salads, 69,
    82
Fruit pie filling, 77
Fruit salad, 57, 97
Fruit shake, 88

Game meat sauce, 51
Garnishes:
    marjoram, 56
    minced basil, 56
    mint, 56
    sesame cream, 95
    sesame nut, 95
    See also Salad dressings;
        Sauces
Gelatin dessert, 45
Gnocchi, 58
Granola, 52
Grape pie filling, 54
Ground oats pie crust, 54
Guinea hen, sesame, 91

Honey sauce for puddings, 93

Ice cream:
    banana, 65
    nut sundae, 65
Italian dressing, 93

Jam, dried fruit, 67
Jerusalem artichokes, 81

Legumes, 96. See also
        Vegetables
Lentil soup, 98
Lima bean pudding, 98

Marjoram, 56
Marjoram milk, 47
Mayonnaise:
    blender, 94
    mayonnaise #2, 94
Meat(s):
    beef, 48, 51
    chicken, 91, 92
    meat loaf, basic, 47
    pork, 78
    rabbit, 78, 79

turkey, 66
veal loaf, jellied, 48
See also Fish; Fowl
Meatballs, 49
Meat loaf, basic, 47
Meat sauces:
    game, 51
    spaghetti, 49
Milkshake, 47
Mint garnish, 56
Molasses butter, 56
Molasses crisps, 45
Molasses mounds, 45
Muffins:
    rolled oat, 41
    rye, 41
    See also Biscuits; Crackers

New Hampshire bannock, 58
Noodles, peanut, 96
Nut cookies, 88
Nut pastry pie crust, 54
Nut squares, 88

Oatmeal sheet bread with nuts, 43
Oat muffins, rolled, 41
Oat waffles, 52
Oil pie crust, 55
Okra:
    boiled, 97
    sautéed, 97
    steamed, 97
Olive oil dressing, 68
Orange flavoring, 93
Orange peel, candied, 86

Pancakes:
    almond arrowroot, 66
    buckwheat, 80–81
    carob, 92
    potato, 53
    rice, 53
    See also Waffles
Peanut butter, 94
Peanut butter cookies, 88
Peanut crackers, 86
Peanut noodles, 96
Peanut waffles, 92